STROKE CERTIFICATION STUDY GUIDE FOR NURSES

Kathy J. Morrison, MSN, RN, CNRN, SCRN, FAHA, is a certified neuroscience nurse, a certified stroke nurse, a Fellow of the American Heart Association, and a recipient of the prestigious Pennsylvania State Nightingale Award for Clinical Nursing Excellence. As the stroke program manager for the Penn State Hershey Medical Center, she oversees all aspects of stroke care, from prehospital through stroke clinic follow-up. She played a pivotal role in Penn State Hershey Medical Center's attainment of The Joint Commission Comprehensive Stroke Center certification and has mentored many stroke program coordinators through the process of attaining Primary and Comprehensive Stroke Center certification. Ms. Morrison serves on The Joint Commission Expert Panel for Stroke Center certification standards.

Ms. Morrison's published works have appeared in nursing journals and neuroscience course curricula. Her book, *Fast Facts for Stroke Care Nursing,* has been well received in the nursing community, both as a handy guide for stroke care nurses and as a preparation tool for the SCRN® certification exam. In addition to speaking nationally on stroke-related topics, she is active in community stroke screenings and awareness lectures and facilitates a regional stroke survivor support group. She established the Stroke Coordinators of Pennsylvania (SCoPA) in 2010—a group of stroke coordinators whose collaborative work has resulted in significant improvements in stroke care and outcomes in community hospitals across central Pennsylvania. She is a Fellow of the American Heart Association, a member of the American Heart Association Professional Education Committee and Hospital Accreditation Science Committee, a member of the American Association of Neuroscience Nurses Advocacy Committee, and a board member of the Susquehanna Valley Chapter of the American Association of Neuroscience Nurses.

STROKE CERTIFICATION STUDY GUIDE FOR NURSES

Q&A Review for Exam Success

Kathy J. Morrison, MSN, RN, CNRN, SCRN, FAHA

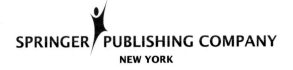

SPRINGER PUBLISHING COMPANY
NEW YORK

Springer Publishing Company, LLC
11 West 42nd Street
New York, NY 10036
www.springerpub.com

Acquisitions Editor: Elizabeth Nieginski
Senior Production Editor: Kris Parrish
Compositor: Exeter Premedia Services Private Ltd.

ISBN: 978-0-8261-1963-6
e-book ISBN: 978-0-8261-1966-7

21 22 23 24 / 10 9 8 7

The author and the publisher of this Work have made every effort to use sources believed to be reliable to provide information that is accurate and compatible with the standards generally accepted at the time of publication. Because medical science is continually advancing, our knowledge base continues to expand. Therefore, as new information becomes available, changes in procedures become necessary. We recommend that the reader always consult current research and specific institutional policies before performing any clinical procedure. The author and publisher shall not be liable for any special, consequential, or exemplary damages resulting, in whole or in part, from the readers' use of, or reliance on, the information contained in this book. The publisher has no responsibility for the persistence or accuracy of URLs for external or third-party Internet websites referred to in this publication and does not guarantee that any content on such websites is, or will remain, accurate or appropriate.

Library of Congress Cataloging-in-Publication Data

Names: Morrison, Kathy (Nurse), author
Title: Stroke certification study guide for nurses: Q&A review for exam
    success / Kathy J. Morrison.
Description: New York, NY: Springer Publishing Company, LLC, [2017]
Identifiers: LCCN 2017004914 I ISBN 9780826119636 I ISBN 9780826119667 (e-book)
Subjects: I MESH: Stroke—nursing I Examination Questions
Classification: LCC RC388.5 I NLM WY 18.5 I DDC 616.8/10076—dc23
LC record available at https://lccn.loc.gov/2017004914

Contact us to receive discount rates on bulk purchases.
We can also customize our books to meet your needs.
For more information please contact: sales@springerpub.com

Printed in the United States of America.

Contents

CONTENTS

Contributor

Alicia M. Richardson, MSN, RN, ACCNS-AG, Stroke Program Clinical Nurse Specialist, Penn State Hershey Medical Center, Hershey, Pennsylvania

Preface

Stroke care nurses have known for a long time that a specialized body of knowledge and a specific skill set are involved in the complex care needs of their stroke patients. Over the past 15 to 20 years, nurses who found themselves working with this distinct population (and many did not consciously seek out the challenge) also found the need for collaboration and support from their peers across the country. As research evidence led to practice standards and Stroke Center certification, nurses recognized that a specialty was being born.

This study guide is designed to serve as a comprehensive, but efficient, tool for preparing for the American Board of Neuroscience Nursing's Stroke Certified Registered Nurse (SCRN®) certification. My first book, *Fast Facts for Stroke Care Nursing*, published in 2014, was designed to be a practical, concise guide for nurses caring for stroke patients. I believed that the more nurses knew about this population and the care needed, the more they would embrace their role and realize that neuroscience nursing is not an intimidating field, but an exciting field—the new frontier in nursing. The feedback I received was overwhelmingly positive: I heard from nurses who discovered a passion for stroke care, nurses who utilized the book to help their organization prepare for and attain Stroke Center certification, and nurses who expressed gratitude for a pocket-sized reference that was quick and easy to use. I also heard from many nurses who described the book as a great study guide for the SCRN exam, and they asked me to add practice questions. So, I took that suggestion and created this study guide.

The book's format follows the test content outline. I have provided 300 questions divided into categories. The number of questions in each category fits the percentage of the test dedicated to that category. For instance, the anatomy and physiology (A&P) section is weighted as 12% of the exam, so there are 36 A&P questions (12% of 300 equals 36). I have also included medication tables, a national stroke care guidelines list, and neuroscience terms for quick reference. Case studies are a valuable tool used in nursing education, so I included a chapter of case studies to stimulate some critical thinking and application of knowledge as an additional preparation tool.

If you have any comments or suggestions for this book, or want to contact me, please do so at kmorrison98@gmail.com.

Kathy J. Morrison

I

Background

Although health care professionals have been caring for stroke patients for hundreds of years, the past 15 years have been marked by dramatic changes in the way care is delivered. Seemingly overnight, stroke care changed from essentially a focus on rehabilitation, to being viewed as a true emergency. This time frame coincides with the acceptance of evidence-based practice as the cornerstone of the nursing profession. This convergence of nursing's professional growth and research-guided evidence has ignited a revolution in stroke care nursing. The specialty of neuroscience nursing has been well established for over 40 years, but has shown remarkable growth with the surge of interest in cerebrovascular nursing. Along with advances in neuroelectrophysiology and neuro-oncology, cerebrovascular nursing has contributed to the phenomenon of neuroscience nursing as the new frontier in nursing.

Brief History of Stroke Care

Stroke care nursing is not new; in fact, people have been having strokes for thousands of years. The first time the term "stroke" was noted in English literature to refer to a health condition was in 1689 by William Cole. Hippocrates is credited with coining the word "apoplexy" as far back as 400 BCE to represent episodes of convulsions and paralysis, typically on the opposite side of the body from the side of injury in the brain. He also described episodes of impaired speech, similar to what is known as aphasia today. The ancient Greeks believed that someone suffering a stroke had been struck down by the gods.

Stroke care first appeared in nursing texts in 1890, but only as very brief discussion. The treatment was supportive care and rehabilitation, but only if the patient survived the stroke and avoided the multitude of secondary injuries that could occur.

The World Health Organization defined stroke in 1970 as "rapidly developing clinical signs of focal or global disturbance of cerebral function, lasting more than 24 hours or leading to death, with no apparent cause other than that of vascular origin." This definition is still used today, but an update is needed given the advances in knowledge about the nature, timing, recognition, and imaging of stroke (Sacco et al., 2013).

With the advent of tissue plasminogen activator (tPA), the year 1996 could be considered the watershed moment for acute stroke care. That year the Food and Drug Administration (FDA) approved IV tPA as the first—and still only—medication for the treatment of acute ischemic stroke. The research outcome was that patients who received IV tPA would have 30% better functional outcomes at 3 months than those who did not receive it. The FDA approval of IV tPA has become known as the turning point for acute stroke care. Stroke was now an emergency, a brain attack.

Introduction of the Brain Attack Coalition

The Brain Attack Coalition (BAC) began in 1991 with a group of neurosurgeons who conceptualized improving stroke care through standardization and evidence-based guidelines. The improved outcomes seen with trauma guidelines served as their incentive. The BAC has grown to include membership from 17 professional organizations. This group of highly educated professionals passionate about stroke care reviewed over 600 research articles related to stroke care, and in 2000, published "Recommendations for the Establishment of Primary Stroke Centers" in the *Journal of the American Medical Association*. This publication, coming just 4 years after the FDA's approval of IV tPA, contributed to the buzz that was developing in the more progressive health care organizations around the country: Stroke patients should receive care that had been proven through research to improve outcomes. This meant that hospital organizations had the opportunity and responsibility to support evidence-based practice for stroke care (Box 1.1).

Box 1.1 BAC Member Organizations

American Academy of Neurological Surgeons

American Academy of Neurology

American Association of Neuroscience Nurses

American College of Emergency Physicians

American Society of Neuroradiology

American Stroke Association

Centers for Disease Control and Prevention

Congress of Neurological Surgeons

National Association of Chronic Disease Directors

National Association of EMS Physicians

National Association of State EMS Officials

National Institute of Neurological Disorders and Stroke

National Stroke Association

Neurocritical Care Society

Society of NeuroInterventional Surgery

Stroke Belt Consortium

U.S. Department of Veterans Affairs

BAC, Brain Attack Coalition; EMS, emergency medical services.

Nursing's Leadership Role in Stroke Care

Despite the unfortunate fact that the BAC did not mention the importance of having nurse coordinators to oversee the immense job of implementing evidence-based standards in acute care hospitals, the majority of organizations came to that conclusion sooner or later, and a whole new category of neuroscience nurses was born—stroke program coordinators. The BAC made amends for that omission with their 2005 Recommendations for Comprehensive Stroke Centers. In this they detailed the importance of not only educated and competent bedside nurses, but also the importance of having advanced practice nurses (APNs) as well.

Nursing Certifications

Specialty nursing certification signifies the attainment of a higher level of knowledge and competence in a specific area. Unlike licensure requirements,

3

certifications are optional, although the popularity—and number—of nursing certifications continues to grow. As far back as 1997, Barbara Stevens Barnum wrote, "We are in the throes of a love affair with certification in this country, and virtually every RN has a string of (possibly) inexplicable certification initials following their signature." Certification requirements ensure that continuing education and clinical experience are maintained, a practice proven to raise the level of nursing professional practice. The CNRN (Certified Neuroscience Registered Nurse) established in 1978, and the SCRN® (Stroke Certified Registered Nurse), established in 2013—both by the American Board of Neuroscience Nursing (ABNN)—are excellent examples of stroke-related nursing certifications.

The American Association of Neuroscience Nurses (AANN) and the ABNN recognized that a subspecialty of neuroscience nursing had been born as a result of the research evidence and care guidelines for the complex stroke population. AANN members were asking for more educational opportunities specific to stroke care, and as these nurses developed more expertise and experience, it became clear that there was an opportunity for recognition of that level of knowledge and expertise. The SCRN exam was developed to provide the tool to prove stroke nursing expertise.

Reference

Sacco, R., Kasner, S., Broderick, J., Caplan, J., Connors, B., Culebras, A., . . . Vinters, H. (2013). An updated definition of stroke for the 21st century: A statement for healthcare professionals from the American Heart Association/American Stroke Association. *Stroke, 44*, 2064–2089.

2

About the SCRN® Exam

Certification Exam Overview

The American Board of Neuroscience Nursing (ABNN) is a not-for-profit corporation with the purpose of creating and overseeing programs for certification of professional nurses within neuroscience nursing (www .abnncertification.org).

The American Association of Neuroscience Nurses (AANN) was founded in 1968 with the purpose of advancing the science and practice of neuroscience nursing. It accomplishes this through provision of continuing professional education, information sharing, research support, standard setting, and advocacy of not only neuroscience nursing, but also advocacy of patients and their families (www.aann.org).

These two organizations work closely together for the mutual goal of advancement of stroke nursing certification via the SCRN® (Stroke Certified Registered Nurse) exam. The SCRN certification exam is only available through the ABNN and the AANN. The SCRN certification is valid for 5 years.

SCRN Eligibility Criteria

1. A current, unrestricted RN license in the United States, Canada, or in a United States Territory that utilizes the U.S. State Board Test Pool Exam or National Council for Licensure Exam. Audits to validate current licensure will be conducted. Candidates from other countries must meet comparable

license requirements, and must be able to read and understand English, as the test is administered in English.

2. Status as a professional nurse working in stroke care including bedside (direct practice), research, educator, administrator or consultant (indirect practice)—with a minimum of 2 years of stroke care experience as a registered nurse within the past 5 years. The ABNN indicates that the experience criteria established does not preclude a candidate with less experience from taking the exam.

3. Completion of the online certification application and submission with fee—must be received by ABNN prior to the application deadline.

Questions about eligibility can be addressed by emailing info@abnncertification.org.

Exam Format

- The SCRN exam is a computer-based test (CBT) in a multiple-choice format. Each question has four answer options with only one of the answers being correct. There are 170 questions (20 of which are possible future questions and do not count toward your score), with 3 hours allowed for completion.
- The exam will be automatically terminated after 3 hours. A digital clock is included for tracking time, and this feature may be turned off during the exam if desired.
- The questions are presented one at a time, with the question number appearing in the lower right area of the screen. You may change your answer as many times as you want until the allotted time is exhausted. To advance to the next question, click on the forward arrow in the lower right area of the screen.
- Questions can be bookmarked for later review by clicking on the blank square to the right of the Time button. To advance to the next unanswered or bookmarked question, click on the hand icon.

Exam Categories

The ABNN has based the exam categories and percentage of the total score dedicated to each category on extensive research of stroke and stroke care nursing. The content is divided as follows:

Anatomy and physiology: 12%
Preventive care: 10%

Hyperacute care: 20%
Stroke diagnostics: 10%
Acute care: 25%
Medications: 10%
Postacute care: 8%
Systems and quality care: 5%

Notification of Exam Results

- Exam results will be provided to the test taker upon completion of the exam, and certificates will be mailed to those who achieved the passing score.
- Those who fail the exam may reapply and retake it as often as they desire. The eligibility criteria must be met each time, along with a new application and fee.

Exam Administration

- Examination services are provided by Applied Measurement Professionals (AMP), a PSI business, in contract with ABNN.
- The exam is offered year-round at more than 190 AMP assessment centers across the United States and internationally. Registration at a testing site will be possible after you receive confirmation of the completed online exam application from ABNN. For a list of test sites, see online.goamp.com/CandidateHome/assessmentCenterNetwork Locations.aspx
- The exam is by appointment—Monday through Friday between 9:00 a.m. and 1:30 p.m. Some locations may have evening and Saturday appointments.
- Candidates requesting special accommodations must call AMP at 888-519-9901 to schedule their exam.

Scheduling an Exam Appointment

- Online: www.goAMP.com and select "Candidates."
- By phone: call toll-free 888-519-9901 Monday through Thursday, between 7:00 a.m. and 9:00 p.m. (Central Time), Fridays between 7:00 a.m. and 7:00 p.m., and Saturdays between 8:30 a.m. and 5:00.p.m.
- Be prepared to confirm a date and location for testing, and to provide your name and candidate identification number (from AMP's email scheduling notice).

Rescheduling an Exam Appointment

- You may reschedule your exam appointment **one time** at no charge as long as the new date is within your eligibility window. To do so, call AMP at 888-519-9901 at least 2 business days prior to your scheduled appointment date.

Postponing an Exam Appointment

- If your exam has not yet been scheduled, you may postpone your exam window to the next exam window **one time**; contact AMP: 888-519-9901.

Canceling an Exam Application

- If you have completed the application process, but have not yet scheduled your exam date, and wish to cancel your application, contact ABNN at info@abnncertification.org. Refunds (minus a $100 administrative fee) will only be made for requests received a minimum of 7 days prior to the scheduled exam window.

This information, along with more details, is available at www.abnncertification.org or www.aann.org.

Common Questions About the SCRN Exam

1. Do I have to be a member of AANN to take the SCRN exam?
   Answer: No, nonmembers can take the test. Members receive a discounted exam fee.

2. Is there a penalty for guessing on the SCRN exam?
   Answer: No, there is no penalty for guessing.

3. Can I skip a question and return to it later?
   Answer: Yes, questions can be left unanswered and returned to later during the exam time period.

4. How soon can I retake the exam if I fail it?
   Answer: The ABNN does not specify a waiting period to retake the exam as do some other certifying organizations.

5. What if I do not think any of the answer choices for a question are correct?
   Answer: You will need to make your best guess from the choices provided. Be assured that the test questions have been reviewed by multiple content

experts at AANN. It is possible to post an online comment by clicking on the button displaying an exclamation point to the left of the time button. The comments will be reviewed, but an individual response will not be provided.

6. What is a passing score for this exam?

   Answer: The passing score is determined by a procedure that involves the judgment of national neuroscience nursing experts and professional psychometricians from AMP, the company that administers the exam, so there is no specific passing score. A scaled score is utilized to ensure a consistent scale of measurement, regardless of which exam a candidate was given. In other words, the raw score of a more difficult version of the exam would not equate with the raw score of a less difficult version. So the raw scores are converted to scaled scores for determination of pass or fail.

7. What if there is a snowstorm, hurricane, tornado, tsunami, earthquake, or massive highway closure on the day of my exam and I cannot get to the testing site?

   Answer: The testing administrator, AMP, will determine if circumstances warrant cancellation or rescheduling. Scheduled candidates will be notified regarding rescheduling if this occurs. You can also visit their website at www.goAMP.com for information.

8. Which certification should I pursue, the SCRN or the Certified Neuroscience Registered Nurse (CNRN), or both?

   Answer: This is a personal choice based on professional experience, goals, and employment setting. Neuroscience nurses working in a setting that includes a variety of neuroscience populations, including stroke, might be interested in pursuing both certifications. Stroke is covered on the CNRN exam, but obviously not in the detail that it is covered in the SCRN exam. It might help to understand the distinctions between the two certification exams (see Table 2.1).

TABLE 2.1 Comparison of SCRN and CNRN Exams

	SCRN	CNRN
Year of origination	2013	1978
Number certified	Over 2,250	Over 4,900

(continued)

TABLE 2.1 Comparison of CNRN and SCRN Exams (*continued*)

	SCRN	CNRN
Experience required	2 years stroke care nursing	2 years full-time neuroscience nursing
Duration of certification	5 years	5 years
Cost of certification	Same for both	
Categories covered	Adult stroke–specific	Pediatric and adult neuroscience spectrum
Number of questions	170 (150 count toward score)	220 (200 count toward score)
Testing time	3 hours	4 hours

CNRN, Certified Neuroscience Registered Nurse; SCRN, Stroke Certified Registered Nurse.

Maximizing Your Score

1. Consider attending a review course, if there is one available. Also, consider a group of colleagues who might be interested in studying together for the SCRN certification exam. Each member could outline a different topic to present to the group.
2. A few weeks before your exam date, design a notes sheet that you will memorize right before the exam. Common items might be the cranial nerves, or generic/trade names of important drugs.

The Night Before the Exam

3. Ensure that you have your ID and the test date confirmation information to take along with you.
4. Ensure that you know the route to the testing center, and plan for extra time to get there.
5. Get adequate sleep—avoiding heavy meals and alcohol 3 to 4 hours prior to bedtime is helpful.

The Day of the Exam

6. Arrange for wake-up time that allows you to get ready and eat without rushing.

7. Avoid a heavy breakfast, and try to include a combination of protein and complex carbohydrate for sustained energy.

8. When you start the exam, utilize any time left from the tutorial session, and jot down the notes you have memorized. This often helps you to relax as you know you have those things jotted down now.

9. The first several questions are often some of the hardest. Keep this in mind, and remember to use the feature that allows you to mark a question so you can skip it and come back to it later, after you've gotten into your rhythm with more questions.

10. Familiarize yourself with the generic names of common stroke medications (refer to the list provided in this study guide). The test will only refer to the generic names, so be prepared.

11. If the choices of a particular question do not make sense to you, try reading them in reverse order—the last one first.

12. Sometimes there is more information provided than is needed. Try not to read into the questions or answer choices—take them at face value. If there is a large paragraph, consider reading the last sentence first to get an idea of what they're asking, then read the paragraph.

13. Do not leave any questions unanswered. Remember, there is no penalty for guessing, so you have a 25% chance of being right, which is better than a 0% if you leave it blank.

14. If you find yourself feeling panicky or overwhelmed, consider a quick break. There is no pause in the time window for breaks, so keep it to less than 5 minutes. But a change of scenery, a quick drink, a bathroom stop, and maybe even splashing water on your face may be helpful. Also remember the simple technique of slow deep breaths.

15. When you have finished, take the time to congratulate yourself and your colleagues for having the discipline and focus to prepare for and take this important certification exam.

3

Anatomy and Physiology

QUESTIONS

1. Subarachnoid hemorrhage is most commonly caused by

   A. Aneurysmal rupture
   B. Arteriosclerotic vascular disease
   C. Arteriovenous vascular malformation rupture
   D. Amyloid angiopathy

2. The dural fold that separates the cerebrum from the cerebellum is the

   A. Corpus callosum
   B. Tentorium
   C. Falx
   D. Posterior fossa

3. The innermost meningeal layer that fits the brain like a latex glove fits the hand is the

   A. Dura mater
   B. Arachnoid mater
   C. Central mater
   D. Pia mater

ANSWERS TO THIS SECTION CAN BE FOUND ON PAGE 21   **13**

4. The frontal lobe contains which of the following?

  A. Wernicke's area
  B. Motor strip
  C. Sensory strip
  D. Globus pallidus

5. The postcentral gyrus is located in the

  A. Parietal lobe
  B. Occipital lobe
  C. Pons
  D. Cerebellum

6. Which of the following best describes the homunculus?

  A. Portion of midbrain responsible for being awake and aware
  B. Another name for the large third ventricle
  C. Diagram that represents the optic path from frontal to occipital lobe
  D. Diagram that depicts what body parts are controlled by the motor/ sensory strips

7. The _____ is the relay station between the cerebral cortex and the brainstem.

  A. Thalamus
  B. Hypothalamus
  C. Putamen
  D. Circle of Willis

8. The diencephalon refers to which structures?

  A. Midbrain, pons, medulla
  B. Basal ganglia, putamen, internal capsule
  C. Thalamus, hypothalamus, pineal gland
  D. Thalamus, globus pallidus, caudate nucleus

9. Someone who cannot understand what is said to them has had an infarct of the

  A. Frontal lobe
  B. Occipital lobe

C. Temporal lobe

D. Brainstem

10. Which brainstem structure connects to the spinal cord and controls respiratory and heart rates?

   A. Medulla oblongata
   B. Pons
   C. Midbrain
   D. Cerebellum

11. You are an emergency department (ED) nurse whose patient presented with staggering gait and slurred speech. The patient denies having been drinking and the alcohol level is normal, but the CT scan is positive for an infarct in the

   A. Midbrain
   B. Right parietal lobe
   C. Occipital lobe
   D. Cerebellum

12. The most common cardioembolic source for stroke is

   A. Mitral valve insufficiency
   B. Endocarditis of the tricuspid valve
   C. Atrial fibrillation
   D. Supraventricular tachycardia

13. Which of these is *not* part of the circle of Willis?

   A. Middle cerebral arteries
   B. Internal carotid arteries
   C. Posterior communicating arteries
   D. Posterior cerebral arteries

14. Patients with adequate blood supply around the borders of their infarct zone have good

   A. Communicating circulation
   B. Cerebral perfusion pressure
   C. Collateral circulation
   D. Borderline circulation

15. Which statement is true?

A. The vertebral arteries connect the subclavian arteries and the posterior brain

B. The basilar arteries connect the common carotids with the circle of Willis

C. The posterior cerebral arteries connect to the cerebellum via the posterior inferior cerebellar artery

D. The cerebellar arteries connect the vertebral arteries to the spinal arteries

16. A deep vein thrombosis can cause a stroke only if there is a presence of what cardiac structure?

A. Atrial fibrillation

B. Endocarditis

C. Mitral valve regurgitation

D. Patent foramen ovale

17. Your patient with an anterior cerebral artery territory stroke is acting "frontal." What is the patient doing?

A. Having trouble hearing

B. Exhibiting left arm weakness

C. Behaving inappropriately

D. Seeing double

18. Which syndrome would you think of for a patient who presents with acute right-sided weakness; that is, right facial droop, right arm = 2/5 strength, right leg = 4/5 strength?

A. Middle cerebral artery syndrome

B. Anterior cerebral artery syndrome

C. Internal carotid artery syndrome

D. Lacunar syndrome

19. Which of the following is *not* a lacunar syndrome?

A. Disconjugate gaze syndrome

B. Pure motor syndrome

C. Pure sensory syndrome

D. Dysarthria–clumsy hand syndrome

20. Intraparenchymal hemorrhage is synonymous with

A. Intradural hemorrhage
B. Subarachnoid hemorrhage
C. Intracerebral hemorrhage
D. Intraventricular hemorrhage

21. Ondine's Curse refers to a syndrome characterized by cessation of respiration during sleep owing to failure of the automatic respiratory center in the

A. Medulla oblongata
B. Pons
C. Limbic lobe
D. Thalamus

22. Locked-in syndrome refers to a stroke in which area of the brain?

A. Central occipital lobe
B. Pons
C. Thalamus
D. Right cerebellum

23. Which symptom is characteristic in a patient with damage to the Broca's area?

A. Dysarthria
B. Dysphagia
C. Expressive aphasia
D. Inability to understand instructions

24. The most common cause of intracerebral hemorrhage (ICH) is

A. Extreme hyperthermia causing capillary leakage
B. Extreme hyperglycemia damaging the blood–brain barrier
C. Aneurysmal rupture causing high intracranial pressure (ICP)
D. Hypertension causing arterial wall rupture

25. Which area is affected in patients with extinction, formally known as neglect?

A. Parietal lobe
B. Medial frontal lobe

    C. Occipital lobe
    D. Basal ganglia

26. A stroke between two adjacent cerebral arteries is known as a/an

    A. Lacunar infarct
    B. Watershed infarct
    C. Subacute infarct
    D. Associated infarct

27. Which of the following best describes the cerebral cortex?

    A. Folds of gray matter playing an important role in consciousness
    B. Folds of white matter playing an important role in consciousness
    C. Tracts of white matter playing an important role in autonomic function
    D. Tracts of gray matter playing an important role in motor function

28. The corpus callosum is best described by which of the following statements?

    A. A band of gray matter fibers that facilitates communication between the cerebral cortex and the brainstem
    B. A band of white matter fibers that facilitates communication between the left and right hemispheres
    C. The posterior portion of the petrosal sinus that facilitates drainage between the transverse sinus and the jugular vein
    D. The sixth ventricle present in approximately 20% of the population

29. The vascular wall structure that is impacted by uncontrolled diabetes and uncontrolled hypertension is the

    A. Tunica media
    B. Tunica adventitia
    C. Tunica intima
    D. Tunica lateralis

30. Arteriovenous malformations (AVMs) can result in an hemorrhagic stroke. This is due to which of the following reasons?

    A. Arteries and veins connecting directly rather than the usual route of arteries to arterioles, to capillaries, to venules, to veins
    B. Connection of arteries to veins is underdeveloped

C. Circle of Willis anomalies

D. Arteries and veins become fused as a result of chronic hypertension

31. Name the condition that is related to a hypercoagulable state, but can present as intracerebral hemorrhage (ICH) and is treated with heparinization.

A. Subacute bacterial endocarditis

B. Horner's syndrome

C. Moya Moya disease

D. Venous sinus thrombosis

32. The blood–brain barrier plays what role in an acute ischemic stroke?

A. Disruption results in locked-in syndrome

B. An intact blood–brain barrier provides protection from hyperthermia

C. Disruption allows the influx of inflammatory cells resulting in edema and hemorrhagic transformation

D. Partial disruption results in homonymous hemianopia secondary to optic tract irritation

33. Multiple tiny infarcts in the same hemisphere is a clue to which condition?

A. Binswanger's disease

B. Incomplete circle of Willis

C. Vertebral dissection

D. Carotid dissection

34. Normal cerebral blood flow is 45 to 60 mL/100 g/min. At what flow rate does irreversible brain damage occur?

A. Less than 40 mL/100 g/min

B. Less than 30 mL/100 g/min

C. Less than 20 mL/100 g/min

D. Less than 10 mL/100 g/min

35. Under conditions of hyperthermia, what changes occur in the brain?

A. Increase in metabolic needs

B. Decrease in metabolic needs

C. Mitochondrial suppression

D. Cessation of adenosine release

36. Name the circumstance in which thrombolysis might be administered to a hemorrhagic stroke patient.

    A. There is no circumstance for thrombolysis in hemorrhagic stroke

    B. Small subarachnoid hemorrhage

    C. Intraventricular hemorrhage

    D. Interosseous hemorrhage

3

Anatomy and Physiology

ANSWERS

1. **A** Aneurysms are almost always located in the subarachnoid space, and are the most common cause. Choices C and D result in intracerebral hemorrhage (ICH), not subarachnoid hemorrhage (SAH), and choice B is a risk for ischemic stroke, not hemorrhagic stroke.

2. **B** The tentorium is also called the tentorium cerebelli, and means "tent of the cerebellum," so picture it as a tent over the cerebellum, separating it from the cerebrum. The corpus callosum is a band of fibers that connects the two hemispheres; the falx is a dural fold that separates the two hemispheres; and the posterior fossa is the space where the brainstem and cerebellum lie.

3. **D** There are three layers of the meninges, the membrane covering the brain. The outermost layer is the dura mater, the middle layer is the arachnoid mater, and the innermost layer is the pia mater. There is no such thing as a central mater.

4. **B** The motor strip is located at the back of the frontal lobe. Wernicke's area is located at the junction of the temporal and parietal lobes; the sensory strip—although it lies right next to the motor strip—is located at the front of the parietal lobe; the globus pallidus is in the basal ganglia, a subcortical structure.

5. *A* The postcentral gyrus is where the sensory strip lies—in the parietal lobe.

6. *D* The homunculus comes from the a 16th century alchemist's description of a "little man" and this term has been used to describe the pattern of the motor and sensory control of the body.

7. *A* The thalamus relays auditory, somatosensory, visual, and gustatory signals between the cortex and the brainstem structures.

8. *C* The thalamus, hypothalamus, and pineal gland are collectively referred to as the diencephalon, which relays sensory information among brain regions and controls many autonomic functions of the peripheral nervous system.

9. *C* The temporal lobe is where Wernicke's area is. It is responsible for receptive speech. Someone with damage to this area might have trouble understanding spoken or written language.

10. *A* The medulla oblongata is sometimes called the extension of the spinal cord within the skull. It controls heart rate and respiration; without its proper function, we cannot survive.

11. *D* The cerebellum is responsible for coordination and balance. When damaged, it can produce symptoms that have been mistaken for inebriation.

12. *C* Atrial fibrillation is a common cause of stroke because it can result in clots forming in the "quivering" atria; these clots can flow through to the cerebral circulation. Endocarditis can produce emboli, but the tricuspid valve is located in the right side of the heart, and any emboli formed there would flow to the pulmonary system, not to the cerebral circulation.

13. *A* The middle cerebral artery is connected to the circle of Willis, but is not considered to be part of it. The components of the circle of Willis are the internal carotid arteries, the anterior cerebral arteries, the anterior communicating artery, the posterior cerebral arteries, and the posterior communicating arteries.

14. *C* Collateral circulation refers to the "detoured" circulation via small vessels that circumvent a blocked larger vessel.

15. *A* The vertebral arteries connect the subclavian arteries to the posterior brain via the basilar artery.

16. *D* A deep vein thrombosis (DVT), if it becomes mobile, will flow into the right side of the heart via the vena cava. Blood from the right atria passes through the right ventricle, and flows out the pulmonary artery to the lungs, so most DVTs cause pulmonary embolus (PE). A patent foramen ovale (PFO) is an opening between the two atria. If this is present, the DVT can enter the right atrium and pass through the PFO into the left atrium, then through the left ventricle and out the aorta where it can get into the carotid circulation and into the cerebral circulation causing a stroke.

17. *C* The frontal lobe is responsible for many things—motor function, problem solving, spontaneity, memory, language, initiation, judgment, impulse control, and social and sexual behavior. Damage to the frontal lobe can result in inappropriate behavior, often sexual in nature.

18. *A* Middle cerebral artery (MCA) syndrome is characterized by motor and sensory loss in the face, arm, and, to a lesser degree, the leg, on the contralateral (opposite) side of the infarct.

19. *A* Lacunar syndromes are small infarcts of territories supplied by a penetrating artery branch of one of the major cerebral arteries. The area involved is small with finite impact on function. Pure motor syndromes produce only motor symptoms; pure sensory syndromes produce only sensory symptoms; and dysarthria–clumsy hand syndromes produce dysarthria and mild hand weakness. There is no such thing as a dysconjugate gaze syndrome.

20. *C* Intraparenchymal hemorrhage refers to blood within the brain or parenchymal tissue. Intracerebral hemorrhage refers to the same thing, thus is synonymous with intraparenchymal hemorrhage. Intradural hemorrhage is between the layers of the meninges, so not within the brain tissue; subarachnoid hemorrhage is under (sub) the arachnoid mater, between the arachnoid mater and the pia mater; intraventricular hemorrhage is blood in the ventricles, which may have come from either a subarachnoid hemorrhage or an intracerebral hemorrhage.

21. *A* The medulla is the lowest portion of the brainstem and controls respiration, and without its proper function, we cannot survive.

22. **B** The pons is located between the midbrain and medulla and serves as a communication and coordination center between the cerebrum and the cerebellum. Damage results in paralysis in the body and most of the facial muscles, but consciousness remains and the ability to perform certain eye movements is preserved.

23. **C** Broca's area controls motor speech, so damage would result in an inability to speak in meaningful ways, or to use words to express your thoughts correctly.

24. **D** Intracerebral hemorrhage is most commonly caused by arterial rupture due to hypertension; aneurysms are most commonly found in the subarachnoid space, so rupture would result in subarachnoid hemorrhage.

25. **A** The parietal lobe is responsible for proprioception, the interpretation of the position of the body within its environment. Right parietal lobe damage can result in extinction, which is the inability to be aware of the contralateral side of the body in relation to the environment.

26. **B** Watershed infarct refers to stroke in the watershed territory—the space between two adjacent cerebral arteries—which is supplied by tiny penetrating vessels that are the first to collapse in the setting of hypoperfusion.

27. **A** The cerebral cortex is comprised of gray matter. There is no such thing as gray matter tracts, there are only white matter tracts.

28. **B** The corpus callosum is a band of white matter fibers that connects the left and right cerebral hemispheres.

29. **C** The tunica intima is the innermost layer of the arterial blood vessels. Its surface becomes roughened in the setting of uncontrolled hypertension and uncontrolled diabetes, resulting in the vicious cycle of platelet aggregation as the platelets attempt to smooth out the roughened areas. As long as the risk factor remains, the cycle continues and atherosclerosis and arteriosclerosis develop.

30. **A** AVMs are direct connections between arteries and veins that are not normal in human anatomy. The normal blood flow path is from arteries to arterioles to capillaries to venules, and finally to veins. Arteries have

muscular walls to handle the pulsing blood as it is pumped from the heart, but veins do not have muscular walls. Therefore if arterial blood flows directly into a vein via an AVM, the veins are likely to rupture under the pressure.

31. **D** Venous sinus thrombosis is the presence of a clot in the venous sinuses, blocking drainage from the brain. Congestion results in infarction, and often petechial hemorrhage.

32. **C** The blood–brain barrier, when intact, protects against influx of inflammatory cells. When disrupted, this protective mechanism may be incapacitated, resulting in edema and possible hemorrhagic transformation.

33. **D** Carotid dissection is the tearing of the intima of the carotid artery. Commonly, tiny clots form along the torn, rough edges of the tear. As they break off and migrate up to the brain, multiple tiny infarcts can occur, and because each carotid supplies only one side of the brain, dissection would result in infarcts on only one side. In vertebral dissection, the clots that break off and migrate would be joined in the basilar artery, which does not supply the hemispheres—it supplies the posterior brain. Binswanger's disease is a condition of insufficient blood supply to the subcortical tissue, not the hemispheres.

34. **D** At cerebral blood flow values of less than 10 mL/100 g/min, irreversible damage occurs as cellular membrane integrity is lost, calcium flows freely into the cell, and neuronal cell death occurs (Alexander, 2013, p. 19).

35. **A** Under conditions of hyperthermia, metabolic needs increase as individual cells attempt to maintain ionic balance (Alexander, 2013, p. 23).

36. **C** In up to half of the cases of intracerebral hemorrhage, blood spreads into the ventricles where clots can obstruct the internal ventricular system, resulting in hydrocephalus. Research evidence indicates some benefit from infusing tissue plasminogen activator (tPA) into the ventricles to dissolve the clots.

Reference

Alexander, S. (Ed.). (2013). *Evidence-based nursing care for stroke and neurovascular conditions.* Ames, IA: Wiley-Blackwell.

4

Preventive Care

QUESTIONS

1. Which is true of a male patient with atrial fibrillation (a-fib) who scores 3 on either the $CHADS_2$ (congestive heart failure, hypertension history, age ≥75, diabetes, stroke history) or the CHA_2DS_2-VASc (congestive heart failure, hypertension, age ≥75, diabetes, stroke history, vascular disease, age 65–74, sex category) scores?

   A. He had a history of heart failure and diabetes
   B. He should receive an oral anticoagulant
   C. He only needs an oral antithrombotic
   D. He is at high risk of bleeding with an anticoagulant

2. A primary care provider (PCP) who initiates a statin medication for a patient whose medical history includes type 2 diabetes and hypertension would be providing what type of stroke care?

   A. Secondary prevention
   B. Tertiary prevention
   C. Primary prevention
   D. Primordial prevention

3. Your 78-year-old transient ischemic attack (TIA) patient was told by the neurologist on rounds that the patient should consider carotid endarterectomy (CEA) for the left carotid artery stenosis of 80%. The patient is

concerned because there were never any prior symptoms and does not like the idea of surgery on the neck. Your best response would be:

    A. To provide education that research supports this intervention for patients with higher than 70% stenosis and risk factors for stroke (the recent TIA)

    B. To provide active listening, and then offer a second opinion from another provider

    C. To calculate the patient's $ABCD_2$ (age [≥60], blood pressure, clinical features of TIA, duration, and diabetes) score and notify the patient that the score is only 5

    D. To reassure the patient that the neck incision is nearly invisible within 5 years

4. You have a family history of atrial fibrillation on your mother's side. She is turning 60 in a few weeks, and asks you how she can do a self-assessment for atrial fibrillation. What will you include in your response?

    A. The importance of regular visits to the neighborhood pharmacy for blood pressure (BP) checks

    B. Instructions on checking a radial pulse for rate and rhythm regularity

    C. Deep breathing strategies to regulate heart rhythm

    D. Instructions on monitoring for persistent cough and dyspnea

5. You are providing discharge education for your 30-year-old female transient ischemic attack (TIA) patient. Her workup has not revealed a clear etiology for the TIA. Which of the following scenarios would be *most* concerning to you?

    A. She indicates that she occasionally has 3 to 4 beers a day, especially on the weekend, and she is a 1 pack-per-day smoker

    B. Her husband asks if he needs to stop smoking marijuana in the same room as her now

    C. Her history includes that she takes a birth control pill and she is 1 pack-per-day cigarette smoker

    D. She asks you if she will need to take aspirin for the rest of her life because she hates feeling like an old lady

6. In reviewing stroke risk factors at a community health fair, one of the audience members says he has a 20-year history of cigarette smoking. What will you include in your response to the group?

    A. Smoking cessation may not help him anymore, but he has a responsibility to those around him

B. Smoking cessation will eliminate all risk of stroke

C. Smoking filtered cigarettes reduces the risk of stroke by 50%

D. Smoking cessation can result in rapid reduction in stroke risk

7. The international case-control study, the INTERSTROKE study, has found that 10 potentially modifiable risk factors account for what percent of stroke risk?

A. 90%

B. 80%

C. 70%

D. 60%

8. Stroke incidence has remained steady at 800,000 new and recurrent strokes/year, despite the decrease in stroke among people aged 65 to 84 years. Which age group has shown a 44% increase in stroke incidence?

A. Ages 85 to 98 years

B. Ages 50 to 64 years

C. Ages 12 to 18 years

D. Ages 25 to 44 years

9. Over the decade 1998 through 2008, the rate of first stroke among people over age 65 years decreased by 30% to 40%. Increased use of which two treatments has been credited with contributing to this decline?

A. Tissue plasminogen activator (tPA) and mechanical clot retrieval

B. Statins and antihypertensive medications

C. Statins and diabetes medications

D. Antithrombotics and statins

10. All of the following are nonmodifiable risk factors for stroke except which one?

A. Age

B. Gender

C. Atrial fibrillation

D. Race/ethnicity

11. Which racial group has a higher incidence of, and mortality from, stroke because of a higher prevalence of hypertension, obesity, and diabetes?

A. Hispanic/Latino Americans

B. Blacks

C. Whites

D. Native Americans

12. As a nurse providing community education about stroke risk, you hear a woman say that her father had a stroke at age 50 years and she wonders if this increases her risk of stroke. You base your response on what knowledge?

A. There has been no genetic link to stroke risk

B. A parental history of stroke before age 65 years increases stroke risk by 0.1%

C. A positive family history of stroke increases risk of stroke by 30%

D. A subtle connection has been found if stroke was due to hypertension

13. Which is true of stroke risk related to high cholesterol?

A. Each 1% reduction in total cholesterol is associated with a 0.8% reduction in risk of stroke

B. Only high-intensity therapy along with fibrates is effective in reducing stroke risk

C. The beneficial effect of statins is due to their capacity to double the blood–brain barrier

D. There is a direct correlation between the level of cholesterol and risk of mortality

14. The American Heart Association (AHA) guidelines for physical activity to reduce stroke risk include:

A. Moderate to vigorous aerobic activity daily for a minimum of 40 minutes/day

B. Moderate aerobic activity for a minimum of 60 min/day, twice a week

C. Vigorous aerobic activity for 20 minutes, twice a day, three times a week

D. Moderate to vigorous aerobic activity for a minimum of 40 minutes/day, three to four times a week

15. Which of the following combination therapies is thought to provide the most effective primary prevention of stroke among people with diabetes?

A. Tight control of hypertension and statin therapy

B. Glycemic control and antithrombotic therapy

C. Physical activity and glycemic control

D. Physical activity and antithrombotic therapy

16. Of the following patients with cryptogenic stroke, which would you suspect the etiology to be undiagnosed atrial fibrillation?

A. 45-year-old female

B. 85-year-old female

C. 64-year-old male

D. 40-year-old male

17. What is the distinction between secondary prevention strategies for stroke patients versus transient ischemic attack (TIA) patients?

A. Blood pressure control is not as critical for TIA patients

B. Intensive statin therapy is recommended for large vessel stroke patients only

C. TIA patients do not need follow-up

D. Prevention strategies are the same for both stroke and TIA

18. Your patient's wife tells you that she dreads the time that he will be allowed to come home from the acute rehabilitation hospital. She says that all of the information she has been getting is overwhelming, and what she really thinks she will need is advice and support after he is home. How can you help her?

A. Communicate her concerns to the care team and ensure that a community resource guide is provided

B. Familiarize yourself with the resource guide in order to be able to reinforce the information and to supplement with other resources

C. Provide her with information about a local or online stroke support group

D. All of the above

19. Your multidisciplinary stroke oversight team has determined that community education about stroke will be a goal for the coming year. What information will be most helpful in developing a strategic plan for this outreach education?

A. Demographic information of the region, such as race, age, and socioeconomic status

B. The number of stroke flyers that can be produced

    C. The number of nurses/health care members interested in participating

    D. The number of stroke survivors in the region

20. In what circumstance would you expect a right-sided carotid artery stenosis to be treated with a stent rather than an endarterectomy?

    A. When the degree of stenosis is less than 50% and the patient is over age 80 years

    B. When the procedure needs to be performed within 2 weeks

    C. When the degree of stenosis is higher than 70% and there are anatomic or medical conditions present that increase risk of surgery

    D. When the provider who performs endarterectomy is not available

21. Which of the following is true about long-term monitoring for occult atrial fibrillation?

    A. It has been credited with finding 11% more cases of atrial fibrillation than found during hospital stay

    B. It is indicated only for females between 40 and 60 years with cryptogenic stroke

    C. Of the cases found during long-term monitoring, only those with duration over 60 minutes pose risk of stroke

    D. Long-term monitoring involves patients dialing into the control center once daily and holding their finger against the phone speaker for 2 minutes

22. Your transient ischemic attack (TIA) patient has had no other risk factors besides a patent foramen ovale (PFO) revealed on an echocardiogram. The patient expresses concern that the neurologist advised the patient that discharge would be with only aspirin to prevent a stroke. Your response would be:

    A. To suggest a second opinion from another specialist such as a cardiologist

    B. To reassure the patient that research evidence supports this as the best treatment because no deep vein thrombosis (DVT) was found

    C. To explain that you have not kept up on the current evidence so you do not really know

    D. To suggest that the patient ask the primary care provider about it at the follow-up visit

23. Mrs. Mills has intermittent atrial fibrillation and has been on Coumadin for 3 years. She is now your patient in the neuro intensive care unit with an intracerebral hemorrhage. What are the American Heart Association/ American Stroke Association recommendations for safe resumption of anticoagulation in her case?

A. Oral anticoagulation is safe to start for all patients within 1 week
B. Anticoagulation resumption should be held for at least 1 week
C. Low-dose IV anticoagulation should be started within 48 hours
D. Perform an MRI at 24 hours after admission; if stable, initiate oral anticoagulation

24. As your multidisciplinary stroke team is reviewing your organization's stroke education content and process, which of the following is important to keep in mind?

A. Daily reinforcement of education provides better chance for retention of information
B. A fifth- to sixth-grade reading level is recommended
C. Poststroke cognitive deficits or emotional distress will impair patients' and families' abilities to comprehend
D. All of the above

25. Your stroke center serves a community that is predominantly Black (44%), with Whites (32%) and Hispanics (21%) coming in second and third. You have limited personnel resources for community outreach. Which of the following would be the best use of your time/resources?

A. Risk factor screening at the local Crispus Attucks community center
B. Health fair at a local mall involving a dozen other community organizations
C. Health talk at the local senior center
D. Distributing F.A.S.T. cards at a local elementary school

4

Preventive Care

ANSWERS

1. **B** The CHADS$_2$ score is a classification tool for predicting stroke risk in patients with atrial fibrillation. One point is given if any of the following are present: congestive heart failure, hypertension, age above 75 years, diabetes, and stroke or transient ischemic attack (TIA) history (gets 2 points). The CHA$_2$DS$_2$-VASc score can be considered an extension of the CHADS$_2$ scheme by considering additional stroke risk factors that may influence a decision whether or not to anticoagulate. The letters in that acronym stand for the same conditions as in CHADS$_2$, with additional components of: age older than 75 years gets 2 points, so now has subscript 2, vascular disease, age 65 to 74 years, and sex. Patients with a CHADS$_2$ score of 1 receive anticoagulation; males with a CHA$_2$DS$_2$-VASc score of higher than 1 and females with a CHA$_2$DS$_2$-VASc of higher than 2 receive oral anticoagulation (Meschia et al., 2014).

2. **C** Primary prevention seeks to prevent the onset of specific diseases via risk reduction, that is, by altering behaviors that can lead to disease. Primary prevention refers to control of risk factors that already exist in specific populations—people who smoke, people with diabetes, people with hypertension, and so on. Primordial prevention refers to strategies designed to decrease the development of disease risk factors—efforts to

decrease the development of obesity, increase exercise, and provide a well-balanced diet; primordial prevention encompasses the entire population and is not limited to individuals with recognized risk factors. Secondary prevention refers to measures taken to limit risk of another event, such as stroke or transient ischemic attack (TIA). Tertiary prevention refers to efforts to soften the impact of an ongoing illness or injury that has lasting effects by helping to manage long-term, complex health problems in order to improve as much as possible a person's ability to function, quality of life, and life expectancy.

3. *A* The American Heart Association/American Stroke Association guidelines recommend CEA for TIA and stroke patients with ipsilateral (same side as their TIA or stroke symptoms) carotid stenosis of 70% to 99%, and for patients older than 70 years. Patients younger than age 70 would also have the option of carotid artery stent (CAS). Note that choice C is wrong because an $ABCD_2$ score of 5 is a high–moderate score and indicates higher risk of subsequent stroke (Meschia et al., 2014).

4. *B* Knowledge of how to monitor heart rate and rhythm would be the most helpful for someone with a family history of atrial fibrillation, advancing age, but no documented dysrhythmia as yet.

5. *C* While each of these answers may raise an opportunity for lifestyle education, the combination of birth control pills and smoking is proven to be a significant risk for stroke, so that is the most important factor to address.

6. *D* The American Heart Association/American Stroke Association guidelines indicate that "smoking cessation is associated with a rapid reduction in risk of stroke and other cardiovascular events to a level that approaches but does not reach that of those who never smoked," so it is still beneficial for persons to stop smoking even with a long history. There is no evidence of filtered cigarettes reducing stroke risk (Meschia et al., 2014).

7. *A* The INTERSTROKE study provided conclusive evidence that 10 risk factors account for 90% of strokes. "Five risk factors (hypertension, current smoking, abdominal obesity, high-fat diet, and physical inactivity) in the INTERSTROKE study accounted for more than 80% of the global

risk of ischemic stroke and intracerebral hemorrhage. With the addition of five other risk factors, the risk for all stroke rose to 90%. The ten risk factors noted are generally well known but their impact is sobering. Stroke risk reduction begins at a very young age with lifelong adherence to a healthy lifestyle." The other five risk factors are diabetes, excess alcohol intake, increased psychosocial stress, depression, and cardiac causes (O'Donnell et al., 2016).

8. *D* A recently published review of 2000 to 2010 data has shown a surprising rise in stroke incidence in people aged 25 to 44 years. There are multiple suspected causes such as "the rise in the prevalence of type 2 diabetes mellitus, hypercholesterolemia, and obesity that has been observed in high-income countries." In addition, cigarette smoking, alcohol abuse, and illicit drug use are frequent in young people and have tended to increase over time (Bejot, Delpont, & Giroud, 2016).

9. *B* Control of cholesterol and hypertension has been the largest contributor to the reduced incidence of stroke in the older than 65-year age group (Mozaffarian et al., 2015).

10. *C* Atrial fibrillation can be modified—either correction to normal sinus rhythm or rate control and protection from clot formation—with an anticoagulant.

11. *B* In the Atherosclerosis Risk In Communities (ARIC) study, Blacks had an incidence of all stroke types 38% higher than that of Whites. Possible reasons for the higher incidence and mortality rate of stroke in Blacks are a higher prevalence of hypertension, obesity, and diabetes (Meschia et al., 2014).

12. *C* A positive family history of stroke increases risk by 30%. "The increased risk of stroke imparted by a positive family history could be mediated through a variety of mechanisms, including (a) genetic heritability of stroke risk factors, (b) inheritance of susceptibility to the effects of such risk factors, (c) familial sharing of cultural/environmental and lifestyle factors, and (d) interaction between genetic and environmental factors" (Meschia et al., 2014).

13. *A* Even with modest reduction in cholesterol, there is reduced risk of stroke. There is no evidence that addition of fibrates is effective. There is

no evidence of statins doubling the blood–brain barrier. There is no correlation between cholesterol levels and mortality (Meschia et al., 2014).

14. **D** The recommendations are for moderate to vigorous activity 40 minutes/day, three to four times a week. Numerous studies have shown that physically active men and women generally have a 25% to 30% lower risk of stroke or mortality than the least active (Meschia et al., 2014).

15. **A** Tight control of hypertension along with statin therapy has been shown to be the most effective primary prevention strategy for people with diabetes. The role of antithrombotics is unclear (Meschia et al., 2014, p. 3771).

16. **B** While the incidence of atrial fibrillation is not remarkably different between men and women, it is more common in women over age 65 years and women have a higher incidence of stroke as a result of atrial fibrillation than men (Mozaffarian et al., 2015).

17. **D** Prevention strategies are the same for TIA or stroke. Differences lie in whether the event is the first event or a subsequent event, which would trigger intensification of antithrombotic therapy.

18. **D** Support for the caregiver is critical in prevention of readmission to acute care, and for prevention of need for institutionalization. So providing as much information as possible, staying educated about available resources, and communicating to the care team are all important factors.

19. **A** In order to develop an effective and efficient education plan for the community, it would be helpful to determine the demographic makeup so that the focus can be on the highest need areas.

20. **C** Patients with a high degree of stenosis, but have either anatomical (history of neck trauma/scarring) or medical (severe lung disease, cardiac disease) conditions that make surgery risky, are treated with stenting rather than endarterectomy. Patients older than age 70 years are recommended to have endarterectomy.

21. **A** Long-term implantable monitors have been effective in finding 11% more cases of atrial fibrillation in patients diagnosed with cryptogenic stroke. There is no gender difference in effectiveness; the correlation between the duration of the atrial fibrillation and the risk for stroke has

yet to be determined; long-term monitoring does not require daily calls or for a finger to be held against the phone (Kernan et al., 2014, p. 2187).

22. **B** While more studies are needed, the guidelines indicate that the research evidence supports an antithrombotic as treatment for PFO without DVT in patients who were not already on an anticoagulant for another reason (Kernan et al., 2014, p. 2202).

23. **B** For patients who require resumption of anticoagulation therapy because of a comorbid condition, waiting longer than 1 week is considered reasonable (Kernan et al., 2014, p. 2210).

24. **D** For patient and family teaching materials to be most effective, they should be reviewed by the multidisciplinary team and checked for fifth- to sixth-grade level comprehension. This ensures that the majority of patients/families will be able to understand the information. Daily reinforcement will help to make the information more familiar, and monitoring for readiness to receive the information is key to ensuring best retention.

25. **A** With limited personnel and resources, it is wise to focus community outreach efforts on the highest risk population—a strategy that has been recommended by the American Heart Association/American Stroke Association. Crispus Attucks, an African American, was the first American soldier to die in the Revolutionary War. His story has come to represent courage and strength, and many Black community centers have been named in his honor.

References

Bejot, Y., Delpont, B., & Giroud, M. (2016). Rising stroke incidence in young adults: More epidemiological evidence, more questions to be answered. Retrieved from http://jaha.ahajournals.org/content/5/5/e003661

Kernan, W. N., Ovbiagele, B., Black, H. R., Bravata, D. M., Chimowitz, M. I., Ezekowitz, M. D., . . . Wilson, J. A. (2014). Guidelines for the prevention of stroke in patients with stroke and transient ischemic attack: A guideline for healthcare professionals from the American Heart Association/American Stroke Association. *Stroke, 45*, 2160–2236.

Meschia, J. F., Bushnell, C., Boden-Albala, B., Braun, L. T., Bravata, D. M., . . . Chaturvedi, S. (2014). Guidelines for the primary prevention of stroke: A statement for healthcare professionals from the American Heart Association/American Stroke Association. *Stroke, 45*, 3754–3832.

Mozaffarian, D., Benjamin, E. J., Go, A. S., Arnett, D. K., Blaha, M. J., Cushman M., . . . Turner, M. B. (2015). Heart disease and stroke statistics—2016 update: A report from the American Heart Association. *Circulation, 133,* e38–e360. doi:10.1161/CIR.0000000000000350

O'Donnell, M. J., Xavier, D., Liu, L., Zhang, H., Chin, S. L., Rao-Melacini, P., . . . Yusuf, S. (2016). Risk factors for ischaemic and intracerebral haemorrhagic stroke in 22 countries (the INTERSTROKE study): A case-control study. *The Lancet, 376*(9735), 112–123.

5

Hyperacute Stroke Care: Prehospital and Emergency Department

QUESTIONS

1. Emergency medical services (EMS) personnel deliver a patient whose blood pressure (BP) has risen from 188/98 enroute to 226/132 on presentation. You double check the cuff size, position, and retake it, with same results. You can anticipate which orders?

   A. Monitor and notify provider if BP exceeds 240 systolic
   B. Stat continuous infusion of IV calcium channel blocker, with rechecks q 5 to 10 minutes
   C. Stat administration of an oral angiotensin-converting enzyme (ACE) inhibitor, with rechecks every 5 to 10 minutes
   D. Stat administration of single dose IV beta blocker, with recheck in 30 minutes

2. Your patient was brought to the emergency department (ED) by her husband who states that when they went to bed at 10 p.m., his wife seemed fine. He went to the bathroom at 2 a.m. and she was sleeping peacefully, but when he woke up at 6 a.m., he found her sitting on the side of the bed

mumbling something about her arm not working right. What is her last known well (LKW) time?

A. 10 p.m.
B. 6 a.m.
C. 2 a.m.
D. Unable to determine

3. Dysphagia screening is essential because patients with dysphagia are at greater risk of mortality due to

A. Hypoxia secondary to severe coughing
B. Dehydration secondary to inadequate fluid intake
C. Heart failure secondary to tachycardia
D. Pneumonia secondary to aspiration

4. You have taken a job in the emergency department (ED) of a small community hospital that does not have neurology support. During orientation, you are shown how to use the telestroke equipment. In which situation will you be using this equipment?

A. During infusion of IV tissue plasminogen activator (tPA) to monitor for vasospasm
B. For communication with the family in the waiting room that is located on another floor
C. For remote neurology/neurosurgery evaluation and treatment recommendation
D. For quick electronic review of compliance with stroke guidelines

5. The difference between an emergency medical technician (EMT) and a paramedic is

A. An EMT is a volunteer, while a paramedic is a paid employee
B. A paramedic receives roughly 10 times the training hours as an EMT
C. An EMT can start IVs and give injections, while a paramedic cannot
D. A paramedic can do the prehospital severity scale scoring, while an EMT cannot

6. The Golden Hour was first described in what population?

A. Stroke
B. Heart failure

C. Status epilepticus

D. Trauma

7. Which is the goal for length of stay (LOS) in the emergency department (ED)?

   A. Less than 24 hours
   B. Between 3 and 6 hours
   C. Less than 3 hours
   D. Minimum of 1 hour

8. Which action results in shorter time from last known well (LKW) to neurologic evaluation?

   A. Calling primary care provider (PCP) immediately
   B. Driving directly to an urgent care center
   C. Driving directly to the emergency department (ED)
   D. Calling 911

9. Which of the following is not a critical action by emergency medical services (EMS) in acute stroke care?

   A. Establishing last known well (LKW) time
   B. Establishing last medication dose/time
   C. Establishing last time lab work was done
   D. Establishing contact info

10. The primary purpose of emergency medical services (EMS) prenotification of arrival of a suspected stroke patient is to

   A. Allow for mobilization of resources in the emergency department (ED)
   B. Ensure a parking spot in front of the ED
   C. Reduce on-site report time
   D. Facilitate tracking of transport times

11. Which of the following is the most common reason for stroke patients not getting acute stroke reperfusion therapy?

   A. Symptoms too mild/rapidly improving
   B. Delay in symptom onset to arrival
   C. Presentation at a hospital not certified as stroke center
   D. Use of anticoagulants

12. Prehospital notification by emergency medical services (EMS) has been credited with which of the following?

   A. Reduced door-to-imaging time
   B. Reduced door-to-needle time
   C. Reduced interhospital transport time
   D. All of the above

13. Emergency medical services (EMS) should not bypass the closest non–stroke-certified hospital if such diversion would add more than ____ minutes to the transport time.

   A. 30 to 40
   B. 40 to 50
   C. 15 to 20
   D. 60

14. Which of the following is a validated and standardized instrument for prehospital stroke screening?

   A. FAST (Face, Arm, Speech, Time)
   B. LAPSS (Los Angeles Prehospital Stroke Scale)
   C. CPSS (Cincinnati Prehospital Stroke Scale)
   D. All of the above

15. Mrs. Brown's husband came in from milking the cows at 8:15 a.m. and found her unable to move her left arm, and looking bewildered. He called 911 and reported she was fine when he had left the house at 7:00 a.m. He was shocked when a helicopter landed in his yard. Why would the dispatcher have sent a helicopter?

   A. All strokes are air transport level now
   B. They suspected a large vessel occlusion (LVO) from the husband's information
   C. The farm is located 50 miles from the closest hospital
   D. Roads were icy

16. Drip and ship treatment has been significantly increased by

   A. Use of telemedicine
   B. Education of emergency department (ED) providers

C. Reduced cost of tissue plasminogen activator (tPA)

D. Education of emergency medical services (EMS)

17. Which of the following statements is true about the emergency medical services (EMS) system in the United States?

A. Protocols are consistent across all states

B. All prehospital personnel are paid and regulated regarding education and competencies

C. Stroke is a high-urgency call in all areas of the country

D. Most state EMS are divided into regions/districts that function independently

18. The 2005 revision of hospital diagnosis-related group (DRG) reimbursement resulted in what change?

A. Hospitals receive an additional $4,000 to $6,000 reimbursement for patients to whom they administered IV tissue plasminogen activator (tPA)

B. Both hub and spoke hospitals receive an additional $5,000 reimbursement for a patient who got IV. tPA and was transferred

C. Hospitals receive $5,000 increased reimbursement for intracerebral hemorrhage (ICH) patients

D. Hospitals receive $1,000 increased reimbursement for patients with length of stay (LOS) less than 3 days

19. The majority of lawsuits in the United States related to the emergency department (ED) phase of acute ischemic stroke (AIS) care are regarding

A. Hemorrhagic transformation after IV tissue plasminogen activator (tPA)

B. Failure to offer IV tPA

C. Delay in CT scanning

D. Emergency medical service (EMS) transport to wrong hospital

20. Which type of patient is more likely to be misdiagnosed in the emergency department (ED)?

A. Patient younger than 35 years with posterior circulation stroke

B. Patient younger than 35 years with anterior circulation stroke

C. Female older than 35 years with anterior circulation stroke

D. Patient older than 85 years with dementia

21. It has been estimated that each 15-minute decrease in IV tissue plasminogen activator (tPA) treatment delay results in

   A. Higher reimbursement for the provider
   B. Higher probability of successful Primary Stroke Center (PSC) certification/recertification
   C. More stable blood pressure over 24 hours
   D. One month of additional disability-free life after stroke

22. There are 7 Ds in the Stroke Chain of Survival: _____, dispatch, delivery, door, data, decision, and drug. Name the first one.

   A. Directions
   B. Distraction
   C. Detection
   D. Duplication

23. Which diagnostic study would you *not* expect to see done with the stat workup of a 32-year-old female who has arrived 1 hour after onset of stroke symptoms, with a National Institutes of Health Stroke Scale (NIHSS) score 7 (arm weakness and sensory loss, aphasia), and no medical history?

   A. Chest x-ray (CXR)
   B. Head CT
   C. Pregnancy test
   D. Serum electrolytes

24. If two of the three categories of the Cincinnati Prehospital Stroke Scale are abnormal, what is the probability of the patient having an acute stroke?

   A. 40%
   B. 68%
   C. 85%
   D. 97%

25. Which of the following best describes crescendo transient ischemic attacks (TIAs)?

   A. A series of three or more TIAs that occur in succession
   B. TIAs that occur within 24 hours after stroke

C. TIAs that follow a seizure

D. TIAs involving the upper extremities

26. Mrs. Newman, a 71-year-old female arrived at the emergency department (ED) at 9:10 a.m. with resolving stroke symptoms. Emergency medical services (EMS) had reported left facial droop, along with left arm weakness, and last known well (LKW) of 6:30 a.m. Her admission National Institutes of Health Stroke Scale (NIHSS) score was 2, and is now 0 at 15 minutes after arrival. Her medical history includes remote smoking history—quit 35 years ago—and hypertension for which she takes lisinopril 10 mg daily and aspirin 81 mg daily. Her CT was negative and point-of-care (POC) glucose was 89. While the provider is discussing treatment options with her, she develops a facial droop and left arm weakness with NIHSS of 5. What is your next action?

A. Continue to monitor the patient, knowing that it is too late for thrombolysis

B. Mix and administer IV tissue plasminogen activator (tPA) as ordered according to her weight

C. Question the nurse who documented the NIHSS to see if it really was 0 or if there might have been some slight deficit remaining

D. Call in the endovascular team in anticipation of mechanical thrombectomy

27. You are a flight nurse for an air medical transport team, and have just arrived at a certified Acute Stroke Ready hospital to pick up a patient for transport to a Comprehensive Stroke Center for management of intracerebral hemorrhage (ICH). Your assessment and management during the flight will focus on which of the following?

A. Monitoring blood pressure (BP) and titration of antihypertensive drip to maintain systolic blood pressure (SBP) at under 185

B. Monitoring neurologic status and vitals for early signs of rising intracranial pressure (ICP)

C. Monitoring reflexes and cranial nerve signs for early vasospasm

D. Monitoring swallow ability and preparation for early antithrombotic dose

28. Mr. Thome is dropped off at the emergency department (ED) by his wife who then goes to park the car. He is identified in triage as a suspected

acute stroke. It takes another 10 minutes to get the CT scanner cleared, and an IV site established. You realize that this is a perfect example of which of the following?

A. The importance of spouses staying with the patient in the ED
B. The need for a second CT scanner in the ED
C. The need for a closer parking area for spouses
D. Benefit of calling 911 and expediting the acute stroke workup process through prearrival notification

29. You are a nurse in the interventional suite of a Comprehensive Stroke Center and just received a patient from the emergency department (ED) with an apparent large vessel occlusion (LVO) of the middle cerebral artery (MCA) whose blood pressure has risen to 180/90 and pulse oxygen has slipped to 86%; the patient is also becoming restless. Your best next action would be which of the following?

A. Explain the importance of lying still for the procedure
B. Change pulse oxygen equipment
C. Prepare for intubation and sedation
D. Restrain patient's arms and legs

30. Which of the following is *not* an exclusion criterion for the 3- to 4.5-hour extended window for administration of IV tissue plasminogen activator (tpA)?

A. International normalized ratio (INR) over 1.0
B. National Institutes of Health Stroke Scale (NIHSS) score over 25
C. History of stroke and diabetes
D. Age greater than 80 years

31. Which of the following tools is *not* used to evaluate for possible large vessel occlusion (LVO) by emergency medical services (EMS)?

A. RACE (Rapid Arterial Occlusion Evaluation)
B. LVOS (Large Vessel Occlusion Score)
C. VAN (Vision, Aphasia, Neglect) score
D. FAR (Face, Arm, Reach) score

32. Your emergency department (ED) patient has just returned from CT angiography with a diagnosis of aneurysmal subarachnoid hemorrhage

(SAH). When you check the patient's blood pressure (BP), it is 178/86. Your most appropriate next action will be which of the following?

A. Continue to monitor, knowing that 185/110 is the top limit
B. Notify the provider and anticipate an order to administer labetalol 10 mg and repeat once with the goal of lowering the systolic blood pressure (SBP) to under 140
C. Administer labetalol 40 mg for SBP to be over 160
D. Notify the provider and anticipate an order to administer labetalol 10 mg and repeat once with the goal of lowering the SBP to under 160

33. For the acute ischemic stroke patient (AIS) in the emergency department (ED), what is the rationale for keeping the head of the bed flat?

A. To remind staff not to give anything orally until after the dysphagia screen is completed
B. To maximize blood flow to the brain
C. To facilitate rest by limiting visual stimulation
D. To minimize risk of headache

34. The use of supplemental oxygen has been found to be appropriate for which acute stroke patient?

A. All ischemic stroke patients
B. All intracerebral hemorrhage (ICH) patients with intracranial pressure (ICP) higher than 16% and O_2 saturation less than 95%
C. All stroke patients with O_2 saturation less than 92%
D. Only hemorrhagic stroke patients with O_2 saturation less than 88%

35. You work in the Neurovascular Intervention (NVI) suite of a Comprehensive Stroke Center (CSC) and have just received word of two patients coming for possible thrombectomy. Two other cases just finished. Which of the four cases described below would you expect less than optimal outcomes?

A. A 85-year-old male with history of hypertension
B. A 70-year-old female with history of atrial fibrillation and hypertension
C. A 62-year-old with history of heart failure and hypertension
D. A 50-year-old with history of diabetes and hypertension

STROKE CERTIFICATION STUDY GUIDE FOR NURSES

36. One of the most effective ways found to improve prehospital stroke care has been which of the following?

A. Increase in the number of paramedics and emergency medical technicians (EMTs) on each call
B. Stricter blood pressure control measures in ambulances and helicopters
C. Approval of paramedics administering tissue plasminogen activator (tPA) prior to CT in select patients
D. Patient-specific feedback provided to transport teams

37. A 78-year-old woman with a 1-year history of declining memory developed sudden headache and decreased consciousness and collapsed while washing dishes. Imaging revealed a right lobar hemorrhage. The most likely cause is which of the following?

A. Hypertension
B. Cerebral amyloid angiopathy
C. Ruptured arteriovenous malformations (AVM)
D. Trauma

38. Your 58-year-old patient arrived within 3.5 hours of symptom onset and her CT scan shows acute intracerebral hemorrhage (ICH). Her husband has been at the bedside looking at his phone, and after the provider has spoken with him about his wife's scan, he asks when she is getting the drug alteplase. What is your best response?

A. "Where did you hear about that?"
B. "Your wife did not arrive within the timeframe for administering that drug."
C. "Your wife's CT showed that she has bled in her brain, and alteplase is not safe for her case."
D. "Alteplase has been studied for use in some hemorrhagic populations, but your wife's provider doesn't like to do that."

39. A 57-year-old woman presents to the emergency department (ED) 45 minutes after the onset of severe expressive aphasia, right hemiparesis, and hemisensory loss. Her National Institutes of Health Stroke Scale (NIHSS) score is 16. Past medical history is significant for coronary angioplasty and stent placement 4 years ago, and surgery on her left foot 5 days ago. She takes aspirin and clopidogrel. On initial presentation, the patient's blood pressure was 190/100 mmHg and is now 170/90 mmHg. Emergent labs and head CT are normal. The patient's symptoms improve to an NIHSS score of 3—aphasia (1), hemiparesis (1), and hemisensory loss (1). Which of the following is a contraindication to this patient receiving tissue plasminogen activator (tPA)?

A. Current use of aspirin and clopidogrel
B. NIHSS score of 3
C. Recent minor surgery
D. None of the above

40. The Cincinnati Prehospital Stroke Scale includes which of the following assessments?

A. Arm drift, facial symmetry, speech ability
B. Arm drift, facial numbness, dysphagia screen
C. Facial symmetry, tongue symmetry, speech ability
D. Speech ability, arm strength against resistance, forehead symmetry

41. You are transporting a patient whom you suspect has had a stroke. She is unable to say the words she wants to say, making it difficult to communicate with her. Which of the following describe the problem with her speech?

A. Ataxia
B. Aphasia
C. Dysphagia
D. Dysarthria

42. Patient D's head CT shows a small intracerebral hemorrhage (ICH). Which of the following in the patient's medical history is the likely etiology of the hemorrhagic stroke?

A. Atrial fibrillation
B. Hypercholesterolemia
C. Diabetes
D. Hypertension

43. Your 65-year-old female patient is apparently having a stroke. She cannot hold herself in an upright position on the stretcher and has begun to vomit. Which of the following actions would be *most* appropriate?

A. Provide a basin and towel and reassure her that she will be fine
B. Place her in the left lateral recumbent position

    C. Insert an oral airway and lower her head

    D. Suction and notify the respiratory technician to bring a ventilator

44. For a patient with expressive aphasia, which is the best strategy for communication?

    A. Speaking more slowly and loudly

    B. Pausing between sentences to allow time to process

    C. Using sign language

    D. Providing pen and paper

45. All of the following are contributing factors for ischemic brain injury except

    A. Blood pressure

    B. International normalized ratio (INR)

    C. Blood glucose

    D. Body temperature

46. Interruption of cerebral blood flow can be caused by all of the following except

    A. Cerebral embolus

    B. Cerebral thrombosis

    C. Cerebral vasodilation

    D. Cerebral vasospasm

47. Which of the following conditions would be *least* likely to mimic the signs and symptoms of a stroke?

    A. Bell's palsy

    B. Hypoglycemia

    C. Complex migraine

    D. Hyponatremia

48. It is important for prehospital personnel to be educated about transient ischemic attacks (TIAs) because

    A. Although the signs and symptoms disappear in a short period of time, they represent a risk for subsequent stroke

    B. The signs and symptoms may be attributed to another less significant cause and might not be transported with as much urgency

C. Patients may refuse to be transported to a hospital so emergency medical services (EMS) needs to educate the patient about the risks of a TIA

D. All of the above

49. A stroke patient is being transported from a Primary Stroke Center to a Comprehensive Stroke Center. IV tissue plasminogen activator (tPA) was started prior to transferring and is continuing to infuse during the transport. The patient's blood pressure (BP) had been stable but suddenly increases to 190/90 with the tPA still infusing. What is the best action by the transport nurse?

A. Allow the tPA to continue infusing while continuing to monitor the BP

B. Stop the tPA and make note of the time, but take no further action

C. Assess for change in neurological status and notify medical command

D. None of the above

50. Because hypertension is a risk factor for hemorrhagic stroke, why would you not treat a blood pressure (BP) of 190/90 in an ischemic stroke patient in the emergency department (ED)?

A. Aggressive treatment can result in hypotension, which could threaten the penumbra

B. Inability to secure an IV site

C. Aggressive treatment could result in hypotension, which could trigger respiratory arrest

D. Inability to secure consent for aggressive treatment

51. Your emergency department (ED) patient presented with onset 2 hours ago of right arm weakness and numbness, which continues. The patient's lab work is normal and head CT is negative for any acute change. The most likely diagnosis is which of the following?

A. Peripheral neuropathy

B. Carpal tunnel syndrome

C. Acute ischemic stroke

D. Transient ischemic attack (TIA)

52. Why are the southeastern states referred to as the Stroke Belt?

A. They have a higher incidence of stroke due to concentration of risk factors such as diabetes, hypertension, and smoking

B. They have a higher percentage of older people, and stroke occurs most often in older people

C. There is a critical shortage of primary care providers (PCP) in that area, so little primary prevention is accomplished

D. That is where the first stroke care was organized in the mid 1990s

53. When assessing your emergency department (ED) patient, a change in pupil reaction to light is considered a late sign of increasing intracranial pressure (ICP). Which is an early sign of increasing ICP?

A. Decline in consciousness
B. Rising pulse oximetry reading
C. Narrowing pulse pressure
D. Decreased hearing

54. You administered an as-needed dose of labetalol 10 mg IV to your stroke patient (blood pressure [BP] 208/108) and note the time to be 12:35 p.m. At 1:05 p.m., you find the patient to be drowsy and slow to respond; BP is 154/84, right where you want it to be. What is your next action?

A. Document the new BP, and continue on to the next patient
B. Perform further neurologic assessment and notify provider of suspected hypoperfusion
C. Perform further neurologic assessment and document that along with the BP
D. Document the new BP and ask the patient care assistant to help you sit the patient up to help stimulate the patient

5

Hyperacute Stroke Care: Prehospital and Emergency Department

ANSWERS

1. **B** IV antihypertensive is the quick action needed with such a high BP, and checks should be within 5 to 10 minutes; answer D is incorrect because 30 minutes is too long an interval between dose and recheck.

2. **A** The LKW time is the time the patient was awake and normal, so even though the husband was awake at 2 a.m., she was asleep, so there is no way of knowing if the stroke had occurred yet or not. You must go with the time they went to bed; 6 a.m. is the time it was discovered, but not the LKW time.

3. **D** Fifty percent of patients with dysphagia will experience aspiration, and 33% of those who aspirate will develop pneumonia (Hinchey et al., 2005).

4. **C** Telemedicine refers to a two-way audio and video connection between two different locations. In stroke care, it is used to provide neurology/ neurosurgery consult expertise to hospitals that do not have onsite consultants experienced with diagnosing and treating acute stroke (Schwamm et al., 2009).

5. *B* Paramedics receive more education and are able to perform more critical care functions than an EMT. Not all EMTs are volunteers; there are many paid EMTs. Both paramedics and EMTs can do the prehospital stroke severity score (Morrison, 2014).

6. *D* The Golden Hour was first described by R. Adams Cowley, known as the father of trauma medicine, in the 1960s based on his observation that the sooner trauma patients reached definitive care—particularly if they arrived within 60 minutes—the better their chance of survival. The term has come to represent the critical first 60 minutes for many populations (Morrison, 2014).

7. *C* The American Heart Association/American Stroke Association guidelines include recommendation for ED LOS benchmark to be 3 hours or less. The intent is for the patient to be admitted to a stroke unit where staff is specifically educated and trained to meet the needs of the stroke patient (Jauch et al., 2013).

8. *D* It has been proven in numerous studies that the quickest way to get a neurologic evaluation for suspected acute stroke is through the emergency medical services (EMS) system (Higashida et al., 2013).

9. *C* Critical actions by EMS that will facilitate rapid evaluation and treatment do not include knowing the last time the patient had any lab work done (Higashida et al., 2013).

10. *A* Enroute prenotification of the arrival of a suspected stroke is important for the EMS so that the CT scanner can be cleared, and the stroke team can be ready to assess on arrival.

11. *B* Delay in patients getting to the hospital after symptom onset is the most common reason for the medication not being given. Symptoms too mild or rapidly improving is also a common reason, but becoming less so as providers are moving toward the policy of asking the patient if he or she can live with a deficit that is deemed mild by the National Institutes of Health Stroke Scale (NIHSS). As the use of the new oral anticoagulants is becoming more prevalent—and until there are reversal agents for those medications—we see increasing numbers of patients not treated with IV tissue plasminogen activator (tPA) due to oral anticoagulants (Higashida et al., 2013).

12. **D** Prehospital notification by EMS has been recognized as contributing to reduced door-to-imaging, reduced door-to-needle, and reduced interfacility transport times (Higashida et al., 2013).

13. **C** Many states have protocols requiring their EMS personnel to bypass non–stroke-certified hospitals. However, if it adds more than 15 to 20 minutes to the transport time, they should not bypass. This is based on the consideration that the patient should first be evaluated and stabilized and then disposition determination can be made (Higashida et al., 2013).

14. **D** All three tools are validated and standardized tools used by prehospital personnel (Higashida et al., 2013).

15. **C** Many state protocols have wording indicating that if travel and transport time will exceed 30 minutes, air transport should be considered. It is no longer just for interfacility transport.

16. **A** The use of telemedicine brings expert consultants into the community ED and has resulted in a significant increase in the number of patients who receive IV tPA (drip) and are then transferred to a Primary Stroke Center (PSC) or Comprehensive Stroke Center (CSC). Education of ED providers and EMS has shown an increase as well, but not as significant as telemedicine (Higashida et al., 2013).

17. **D** Unfortunately prehospital policies vary from one state to another, and most states even have regional variations. Some prehospital personnel are unpaid—and most are underpaid for the important work they do. There are still some areas of the country where stroke is not a high-urgency call (Higashida et al., 2013).

18. **A** In 2005, efforts to increase the number of patients who were treated with tPA included increased reimbursement to cover the high cost of the drug (Higashida et al., 2013).

19. **B** The majority of lawsuits in the United States related to the ED phase of stroke care are regarding the failure to offer tPA. It is the standard of care and must be made available if the patient qualifies (Higashida et al., 2013).

20. **A** Posterior circulation strokes do not produce such classic symptoms as hemispheric strokes, and are often misdiagnosed, particularly in younger people who are not expected to have strokes (Arch et al., 2016).

21. **D** Based on multiple research study data, it has been estimated that each 15-minute reduction in door-to-needle time results in an additional disability-free life after stroke (Middleton, Grimley, & Alexandrov, 2015).

22. **C** The first D in the Stroke Chain of Survival is detection, as that is essential for the rest of the chain to occur (Jauch et al., 2010).

23. **A** A CXR is no longer a standard part of most acute stroke workups. It is at the discretion of the stroke team to order if they suspect an underlying cardiac or lung problem for which a CXR would be helpful. The guidelines state that if done, it should not delay the administration of tissue plasminogen activator (tPA; Jauch et al., 2013).

24. **C** The Cincinnati Prehospital Stroke Scale includes assessment of facial symmetry, arm drift, and speech. Research has shown that if two of those three are abnormal, there is an 85% chance that the patient is having a stroke (American Heart Association, 2011).

25. **A** Crescendo TIAs is a term used to describe a series of three or more TIAs in close succession. It is considered to be a strong predictor of impending stroke.

26. **B** If the NIHSS returns to 0 and the patient's symptoms have all resolved, and then the symptoms return, that is the new LKW time and the clock starts again.

27. **B** With a hemorrhagic stroke, the most important thing for the transport team is to monitor for signs of increasing ICP; answer A is incorrect because the BP parameter for ICH is 140 systolic or lower.

28. **D** It has been proven in numerous studies that the quickest way to get a neurologic evaluation for suspected acute stroke is through the emergence medical services (EMS) system (Higashida et al., 2013).

29. **C** For endovascular intervention, patients need to be able to lie still. In this situation, they will need to be intubated and sedated, so preparation for that is correct.

30. **A** Consideration of the extended time window for tPA does not involve a specific INR—if the patient is on Coumadin, regardless of INR, they are not a candidate for the extended window (Del Zoppo, Saver, Jauch, & Adams, 2009).

31. D There are numerous tools being used by the EMS across the country to help determine if there is an LVO, which would indicate the need for transport to a Comprehensive Stroke Center (CSC) or Primary Stroke Center (PSC) with mechanical thrombectomy capability. There is no tool called FAR.

32. D For SAH, the goal is to keep the SBP under 160. The first two answers are incorrect because the BP parameters stated are for ischemic and intracerebral hemorrhage (ICH), respectively. Answer C is wrong because the dose of 40 mg labetalol is too high (Connolly et al., 2012).

33. B After an ischemic stroke, swelling produces compression of the surrounding tissue, and facilitation of perfusion to the brain is helped with the head of the bed kept flat.

34. C Evidence-based guidelines indicate that for best oxygenation of the brain, an O_2 saturation of less than 92% should be supplemented with oxygen.

35. A The studies regarding mechanical clot retrieval did not include age over 80 years, and there has been further evidence that advanced age may be an indicator of less-than-optimal outcome.

36. D Prehospital personnel have reported that getting patient-specific feedback on outcomes has provided them valuable information on which to base expectations and accountability. It has also raised the level of interest in stroke.

37. B Amyloid angiopathy is a condition in which there is accumulation of abnormal proteins (amyloid) in the small cerebral arteries. This accumulation weakens vessel walls leading to intracerebral hemorrhage. It is frequently associated with Alzheimer's disease. This patient collapsed before having any possible trauma. It could have been an AVM, but the declining memory was the clue for the correct answer of amyloid angiopathy.

38. C A simple explanation of the fact that alteplase is not appropriate for a bleed—reinforcing what the provider had just told the husband—is enough.

39. D Foot surgery 5 days ago is not an exclusion for alteplase. As it is a compressible site, it is not unreasonable that this patient could get alteplase safely.

STROKE CERTIFICATION STUDY GUIDE FOR NURSES

40. **A** Arm drift, facial symmetry, and speech ability are the components of the Cincinnati Prehospital Stroke Scale. The assessment does not include arm strength against resistance; it is simply the ability to hold the arm up against gravity, and note any drift.

41. **B** The inability to say the words you want to say—whether because of inability to speak, or because of inability to say the correct word—is aphasia. Ataxia is uncoordinated movements. Dysphagia is swallowing dysfunction. Dysarthria is slurred speech.

42. **D** The most common cause of ICH is hypertension.

43. **B** Placing the patient in the left lateral recumbent position is the most appropriate thing to do right away to protect against aspiration. As long as the patient is conscious, an oral airway would not be appropriate. The patient may, in fact, eventually need to be intubated, but there are not enough indicators for that yet.

44. **D** Expressive aphasia is the inability to express, or speak. The only suitable answer would be to provide pen and paper to see if the patient can write, which the patient may not be able to do either with certain types of expressive aphasia.

45. **B** INR is not a contributing factor for ischemic brain injury, but blood pressure, glucose, and temperature are.

46. **C** Cerebral vasodilatation is the expansion of the lumen of the vessels so it would not interrupt cerebral blood flow. A thrombus or embolus would be capable of interruption of flow, and vasospasm can narrow the vessel to the point of interruption of blood flow.

47. **D** Hyponatremia produces symptoms of lethargy, thirst, and confusion, which are not classic for a stroke, so not likely to be considered a mimic. Bell's palsy results in facial droop; hypoglycemia results in confusion and slurred speech; complex migraine can produce symptoms such as hemiplegia, visual changes, and headache.

48. **D** EMS personnel who are educated about TIA have the opportunity to help the patient understand that even if the symptoms resolved, they should still go to the hospital for a workup.

49. *C* Transport personnel should assess for neurologic status and notify medical command, in anticipation of an order for an antihypertensive. Answer A is wrong because it does not involve notification or treatment; answer B is wrong because the nurse simply stopped the tPA, but did not treat.

50. *A* Permissive hypertension in an acute ischemic stroke without tissue plasminogen activator (tPA) allows for systolic BP up to 220 with the intent of ensuring perfusion and avoidance of hypoperfusion. Answer C is wrong because it states that rapid lowering would result in respiratory arrest.

51. *C* Acute ischemic stroke can take several hours to show up on a CT scan, so it would be most likely a stroke, not a TIA with persistent symptoms. Peripheral neuropathy is usually in the setting of other comorbid conditions such as diabetes, and carpal tunnel syndrome would be related to hand use/position.

52. *A* There have been many studies done, and some are ongoing regarding the high incidence and mortality from stroke in the Stroke Belt. Lifestyle factors such as diabetes, hypertension, and smoking are thought to be the cause, but genetics likely plays a role as well.

53. *A* Change in LOC is usually the earliest sign of rising ICP. Rising pulse oxygen is not a sign of increased ICP; pulse pressure would be widening in increasing ICP; decreased hearing can be seen with chronic high ICP as with hydrocephalus, but not with acute increase in ICP (Alexander, 2013).

54. *B* Patients with history of hypertension often have a limited tolerance for "normal" BP. Further neurologic assessment is warranted, along with notification of the provider.

References

Alexander, S. (Ed.). (2013). *Evidence-based nursing care for stroke and neurovascular conditions.* Ames, IA: Wiley-Blackwell.

American Heart Association. (2011). Advanced cardiovascular life support provider manual. Dallas, TX: Author.

Arch, A. E., Weisman, D. C., Coca, S., Nystrom, K. V., Wira III, C. R., & Schindler, J. L. (2016). Missed ischemic stroke diagnosis in the emergency department by emergency medicine and neurology services. *Stroke, 47*(3), 668–673. doi:10.1161/STROKEAHA.115.010613

Connolly, E., Rabinstein, A., Carhuapoma, R., Derdeyn, C., Dion, J., Higashida, R. T., . . . Vespa, P. (2012). Guidelines for the management of aneurysmal subarachnoid hemorrhage: A guideline for healthcare professionals from the American Heart Association/American Stroke Association. *Stroke, 43*, 1711–1737.

Del Zoppo, G. J., Saver, J. L., Jauch, E. C., & Adams, H. P. (2009). Expansion of the time window for treatment of acute ischemic stroke with intravenous tissue plasminogen activator: A science advisory from the American Heart Association/American Stroke Association. *Stroke, 40*, 2945–2948.

Higashida, R., Alberts, M. J., Alexander, D. N., Crocco, T. J., Demaerschalk, B. M., Derdeyn, C. P., . . . Wood, J. P. (2013). Interactions within stroke systems of care: A policy statement from the American Heart Association/American Stroke Association. *Stroke, 44*, 2961–2984.

Hinchey, J., Shephard, T., Furie, K., Smith, D., Wang, D., & Tong, S. (2005). Formal dysphagia screening protocols prevent pneumonia. *Stroke, 36*(9), 1972–1976.

Jauch, E., Cucchiara, B., Adeoye, O., Meurer, W., Brice, J., Chan, Y., . . . Hazinski, M. F. (2010). Part 11: Adult Stroke: 2010 American Heart Association guidelines for cardiopulmonary resuscitation and emergency cardiovascular care. *Circulation, 122*, S818–S828. Retrieved from http://circ.ahajournals.org/content/122/18_suppl_3/S818.full

Jauch, E., Saver, J., Adams, H., Bruno, A., Connors, J., Demaerschalk, B. M., Khatri, P., . . . Yonas, H. (2013). Guidelines for the early management of patients with acute ischemic stroke: A guideline for healthcare professionals from the American Heart Association/American Stroke Association. *Stroke, 44*, 870–947.

Middleton, S., Grimley, R., & Alexandrov, A. W. (2015). Triage, treatment, and transfer: Evidence-based clinical practice recommendations and models of nursing care for the first 72 hours of admission to hospital for acute stroke. *Stroke, 46*(2), e18–e25. doi:10.1161/STROKEAHA.114.006139

Morrison, K. J. (2014). *Fast facts for stroke care nursing: An expert guide in a nutshell.* New York, NY: Springer Publishing.

Schwamm, L., Audebert, H., Amarenco, P., Chumbler, N., Frankel, M., & George, M. G. (2009). Recommendations for the implementation of telemedicine within stroke systems of care: A policy statement from the American Heart Association. *Stroke, 40*, 2635–2660.

Stroke Diagnostics

QUESTIONS

1. What is the only blood test you must have results of in order to safely administer IV tissue plasminogen activator (tPA)—besides international normalized ratio (INR), which is required for patients on Coumadin?

    A. Liver enzymes
    B. Cardiac enzymes
    C. Creatinine to know if CT angiography is safe
    D. Blood sugar

2. Patient X presents to the emergency department (ED) with right-sided weakness and speech difficulty at 10:00 a.m., reporting onset at 8:30 a.m. The CT was unremarkable. The wife says the only medication her husband takes is Coumadin. The international normalized ratio (INR) result is 1.9. What can you expect to do next?

    A. Mix and administer tissue plasminogen activator (tPA) according to the patient's actual weight
    B. Repeat the INR
    C. Continue to monitor vital signs and neurologic checks according to ED policy
    D. Prepare to discharge the patient from the ED

ANSWERS TO THIS SECTION CAN BE FOUND ON PAGE 70

3. Identify the main reason why a CT scan is the first imaging study done in acute stroke.

   A. Most hospitals only have CT scan capability
   B. While not completely reliable, it is least expensive and the one insurance will cover
   C. There is less radiation involved than MRI
   D. CT is fast and reliable in ruling out cerebral hemorrhage

4. The consulting neurologist recommends vascular imaging in order to determine if there is a large vessel occlusion. What test would you expect to see done next?

   A. PET scan
   B. CT angiogram (CTA)
   C. MRI
   D. Transcranial Doppler (TCD)

5. Patient Y presents to your emergency department (ED) at 3:00 p.m. with left-sided weakness onset at 10:30 a.m. The CT software is out of service so a stat MRI/magnetic resonance angiography (MRA) package is done that shows a perfusion–diffusion mismatch. This indicates which of the following?

   A. Presence of salvageable brain tissue, so thrombectomy should be considered
   B. Absence of salvageable brain tissue, so thrombectomy is not an option
   C. Technical error by imaging staff
   D. Presence of an uncommon cerebral anomaly

6. Why is an echocardiogram done during acute hospital stays?

   A. The cause of up to 30% of strokes is cardiac related
   B. It is only required on patients older than 80 years
   C. To rule out incidental cardiomyopathy
   D. All patients with stroke are at risk for cardiomyopathy within 10 years

7. Why would the neurologist order a transesophageal echocardiogram (TEE) after the patient has already had a transthoracic echocardiogram (TTE)?

   A. Patient would not lie still for the TTE
   B. TEE offers superior visualization as there is no impedance from the chest muscles or rib cage

C. Latest guidelines recommend both be done for confirmed stroke patients

D. The neurologist made a mistake and should be reminded that an echocardiogram was already done

8. Your stroke patient has just been ordered to have a video fluoroscopic swallowing exam. What is the provider looking for?

A. Confirmation of successful bedside swallow screen

B. Evaluation of swallowing function

C. Evidence of aspiration

D. Both B and C

9. What further diagnostic tool might be used for a patient with cryptogenic stroke prior to or shortly after discharge from the hospital?

A. Serial cardiac enzymes

B. Genetic mapping

C. Repeat CT in 1 month

D. Implantable cardiac monitor to check for atrial fibrillation

10. Your patient was told that she had a stroke at some time in the past, but she insists she has never had symptoms. How did her neurologist know this?

A. Presence of encephalomacia on CT scan

B. Presence of positive Babinski's sign during neurologic exam

C. Prolonged QT interval on 12-lead EKG

D. Information from the spouse during history taking

11. A patient is brought to the emergency department (ED) by emergency medical services (EMS) with an original complaint of the worst headache of the patient's life, and is sleepy on arrival. You look to your ED colleague and say, "I'll bet you it's a _____."

A. Left middle cerebral artery (MCA) stroke

B. Lacunar stroke in the right basal ganglia

C. Complex migraine

D. Subarachnoid hemorrhage

12. Your patient's CT is negative for blood and there is high suspicion for subarachnoid hemorrhage (SAH). What other diagnostic test might you be told to set up for?

A. Lumbar puncture

B. Repeat CT

    C. Blood cultures

    D. Caloric testing

13. Which diagnostic tool has been proven to not only diagnose and monitor vasospasm in subarachnoid hemorrhage (SAH) but also to predict and enhance IV tissue plasminogen activator (tPA) outcomes?

    A. EEG

    B. Diffusion-weighted MRI

    C. PET scan

    D. Transcranial Doppler (TCD)

14. Your patient has just had a diagnostic cerebral angiography. What are the most common complications you will monitor over the next 24 hours?

    A. Insertion site hematoma, stroke, and adverse reaction to contrast dye

    B. Insertion site hematoma, deep vein thrombosis (DVT), and adverse reaction to contrast dye

    C. Fever, headache, and insertion site hematoma

    D. Vessel wall tear, stroke, and DVT

15. The Brain Attack Coalition set separate standards for door-to-CT scan initiation and results. Which of the following is correct?

    A. Door to CT in 35 minutes, results in 45 minutes

    B. Door to CT in 25 minutes, results in 45 minutes

    C. Door to CT in 10 minutes, results in 45 minutes

    D. No completion standard timeframe; just results within 60 minutes

16. You are a stroke unit nurse and your new stroke patient has arrived from the emergency department (ED) without having a carotid ultrasound done. You call the provider to order one stat. Which would be the correct response by the provider?

    A. "Get a carotid ultrasound done stat"

    B. "A CT angiogram was done that provided carotid imaging"

    C. "The patient has an allergy to contrast dye, so a carotid ultrasound cannot be done"

    D. "Carotid disease is so rare that it is not necessary to do carotid imaging in stroke patients"

17. More sensitive brain imaging has contributed to the change in definition of which of the following?

A. Cerebral edema
B. Acute ischemic stroke
C. Subarachnoid hemorrhage
D. Transient ischemic attack (TIA)

18. You are working on a stroke unit with an assignment of four patients today. On which of them would you expect to see a hypercoagulable work-up?

A. An 80-year-old male with right basal ganglia stroke
B. A 45-year-old female with subarachnoid hemorrhage (SAH)
C. A 28-year-old male with right middle cerebral artery (MCA) stroke
D. A 58-year-old female with lock-in syndrome

19. Which of the following is true of CT imaging?

A. Bone and blood appear white and cerebrospinal fluid (CSF) appears black
B. Substances with increased density appear darker, while substances of less density appear lighter
C. It uses same radiologic technology as MRI imaging
D. Subarachnoid hemorrhage (SAH) classically has a white diamond shape in the center of the brain

20. Which of the following is the recommended initial imaging for suspected subarachnoid hemorrhage (SAH)?

A. MRI scan with contrast
B. Cerebral angiography
C. Noncontrast CT scan
D. CT angiogram

21. Early neurologic deterioration with a decrease in the Glasgow Coma Scale (GCS) score of 2 or more points is a hallmark of which type of stroke?

A. Spontaneous intracerebral hemorrhage (ICH)
B. Infratentorial shift
C. Vertebrobasilar syndrome
D. Basal ganglia stroke

22. The presence of a "spot sign" on a CT angiogram (CTA) and contrast-enhanced CT likely indicates which of the following?

    A. Incidental additional pathology
    B. Presence of contrast within a hematoma and increased risk of expansion
    C. Absence of contrast within a large vessel clot
    D. None of the above

23. Which of the following are early CT imaging predictors of cerebral edema?

    A. Frank hypodensity within the first 6 hours
    B. Involvement of one third or more of the middle cerebral artery (MCA) territory
    C. Early midline shift
    D. All of the above

24. Transcranial Doppler (TCD) ultrasonography has proven to be useful in detecting intracranial vessel abnormalities. Which of the following circumstances will produce the most useful results?

    A. Posterior circulation strokes
    B. Middle cerebral artery (MCA) strokes
    C. Patients with poor bony windows
    D. Moya Moya disease

25. In the hyperacute workup of acute ischemic stroke, what priority would you place on completion of a chest x-ray for most patients?

    A. Immediately following noncontrast CT of brain
    B. Immediately following lab work, prior to EKG
    C. Following CT, lab work, and EKG
    D. Following lab work, prior to EKG

26. The emergency medical services (EMS) personnel report that a 70-year-old male with new onset left-sided weakness is taking dabigatran, an oral anticoagulant. Which blood test will be helpful in determining the effect of this medication?

    A. Prothrombin time (PT)/INR
    B. Partial thromboplastin time (PTT)
    C. Platelet count
    D. None of the above

27. Dr. West, the stroke neurologist, mentions that a malignant middle cerebral artery (MCA) sign was noted on Mrs. Bender's CT. What did the neurologist see?

    A. Malignant tumor in the area of the MCA territory causing mass effect
    B. Ischemic infarct involving more than 50% of the MCA territory with a midline shift
    C. Hemorrhagic infarct involving more than 30% of the MCA territory with a midline shift
    D. Vasospasm of the proximal MCA resulting in 50% reduced perfusion to territory

28. When President Dwight D. Eisenhower had a stroke in 1957, his diagnosis was left middle cerebral artery (MCA) infarct. Which diagnostic test would have contributed to his stroke diagnosis?

    A. Noncontrast CT
    B. MRI
    C. Echocardiogram
    D. None of the above

29. A patient who had a cerebral angiogram this morning has become diaphoretic and is complaining of lower abdominal pain and back pain. You suspect which of the following?

    A. Arterial thrombosis with restricted perfusion pattern
    B. Muscle spasm from prolonged immobility
    C. Arterial dissection with retroperitoneal hemorrhage
    D. Unintentional migration of the closure device

30. Your patient is headed to radiology for a CT angiogram and you do a quick review of reported allergies knowing that the patient will be getting contrast. Which of the following allergies will you immediately report?

    A. Shellfish
    B. Red dye #5
    C. Eggs
    D. Nickel alloy

6

Stroke Diagnostics

ANSWERS

1. **D** The American Heart Association guidelines state that "only blood glucose must precede the initiation of IV tPA" (Class I, Level of Evidence B recommendation). They also state that except for patients without suspicion of bleeding abnormality or thrombocytopenia, not on heparin or Coumadin, and not on other anticoagulants, IV tPA administration should not be delayed waiting for any other lab tests. Patients whose creatinine comes back elevated will have a decision made on an individual-case basis as to whether to stop the tPA, or continue (Jauch et al., 2013).

2. **C** An INR of greater than 1.7 is a contraindication for administration of IV tPA.

3. **D** CT scans are more readily available in the majority of hospitals, are significantly quicker, and are reliable in ruling out hemorrhage.

4. **B** CTA is the most frequent emergent imaging test to visualize blood vessels. The prefix *angio* refers to blood vessels, so anytime you see *angio* in the name of a radiologic test it indicates that there will be evaluation of blood vessels. A plain CT looks at brain tissue, and a CTA looks at the cerebral vessels. An MRI looks at brain tissue, and a magnetic resonance

angiography (MRA) looks at cerebral vessels. A PET scan is used to detect cancer, and a TCD is used to detect vasospasm and measure the velocity of the blood flow in the major cerebral arteries.

5. *A* Perfusion–diffusion mismatch has been used in acute stroke to determine presence or absence of salvageable tissue. The difference between the diffusion (water content) of the tissue and perfusion (blood supply) abnormalities provides a measure of the ischemic penumbra, or salvageable tissue. If the perfusion abnormality is larger than the area of restricted diffusion, the difference identifies the region of reversible ischemia.

6. *A* The cause of up to 30% of ischemic strokes is cardiac problems, so an echocardiogram is an essential component of acute stroke workup.

7. *B* For patients with a high suspicion of a cardiac source, or if an abnormality was seen on the TTE that the provider wants to examine more closely, a TEE is used because it is not impeded by the structures of chest muscles or rib cage. It is superior at identifying atrial and aortic abnormalities, such as patent foramen ovale (PFO) or aortic arch atherosclerosis.

8. *D* A video fluoroscopic swallowing exam involves having the patient swallow contrast material while a visualization is done with fluoroscopic equipment. This provides information about swallowing ability as well as evidence of aspiration.

9. *D* For patients with a cryptogenic stroke (unknown cause), evidence has shown that implantable monitors detected atrial fibrillation during the months after discharge in up to 12% of patients who did not have atrial fibrillation detected on standard Holter monitor.

10. *A* Encephalomacia is described as "softening of the brain tissue" and has numerous causes, one of which is stroke. It has a characteristic appearance on CT, and is also referred to as scar tissue after stroke.

11. *D* Subarachnoid hemorrhage patients often have a classic presentation of thunderclap headache, often called "the worst headache of their life." This is thought to be due to the irritation by the blood, increased pressure, and vasospasm.

12. *A* If CT is negative in a patient with a high suspicion for SAH, lumbar puncture will provide evidence whether or not there is xanthochromia in the cerebrospinal fluid (CSF).

13. *D* TCD studies done during infusion of IV tPA to monitor for vessel patency were found to augment the effect of the tPA, supposedly via the effect of ultrasound waves on the clot—it can hasten the dissolution of the clot.

14. *A* Common complications associated with diagnostic cerebral angiography are insertion site hematoma, stroke, and adverse reaction to dye. As this test is done via an artery, DVT would not be a complication.

15. *B* The Brain Attack Coalition's recommendations for timeframes for CT are initiation in 25 minutes and interpretation in 45 minutes.

16. *B* CT angiography provides carotid vessel imaging superior to standard carotid ultrasound, making it generally unnecessary to do a carotid ultrasound during the acute workup (Jauch et al., 2013, p. 885).

17. *D* Improved CT and MRI imaging has made it possible to see even miniscule infarcts. Today, events lasting less than 24 hours, with normal imaging, formerly labeled TIA, are often found to be tiny strokes (Kernan et al., 2014, p. 2166).

18. *C* Young people with large vessel ischemic strokes whose workups are negative for cardiac abnormality often get a set of lab tests that evaluate for a hypercoagulable state, or an abnormal tendency to form clots (Kernan et al., 2014, p. 2204).

19. *A* On CT, blood and bone appear white because they absorb x-rays better than the water content of CSF, which appears black; brain tissue is intermediate in its absorption, so it appears gray (Alexander, Gallek, Presciutti, & Zrelak, 2012, p. 11).

20. *C* Noncontrast CT is the cornerstone of the diagnostic workup for SAH (Connolly et al., 2012, p. 1718).

21. *A* More than 20% of ICH patients will experience a decrease in GCS of 2 or more points (Hemphill et al., 2015, p. 2034).

22. *B* The identification of patients at risk of ICH expansion is based on the presence of contrast within the hematoma on CTA (Hemphill et al., 2015, p. 2036).

23. **D** Predictors of cerebral edema are early frank hypodensity on CT, involvement of one third or more of the MCA territory, and early midline shift (Wijdicks et al., 2014, p. 1228).

24. **B** As TCD is done through the temporal bony window, the MCA and anterior cerebral artery (ACA) can be monitored, but not the posterior circulation (Jauch et al., 2013, p. 885).

25. **C** Chest x-ray may be useful if specific additional conditions such as cardiac or pulmonary disease exist, but it should not be prioritized or delay administration of IV tissue plasminogen activator (tPA; Jauch et al., 2013, p. 881).

26. **D** There are no specific lab tests to measure the effect of dabigatran (Jauch et al., 2013, p. 881).

27. **B** Malignant MCA infarction is a devastating condition, with up to 80% mortality. The pathophysiology is a large core of severe ischemia involving over 50% of MCA territory and only a relatively small rim of penumbra. Cytotoxic edema occurs immediately in a large portion of the ischemic territory. The subsequent damage leads to the breakdown of the blood–brain barrier and vasogenic brain edema, resulting in space-occupying brain swelling. The progressive vasogenic edema reaches its maximum after 1 to several days and exerts a mechanical force on surrounding tissue structures leading to a midline shift and transtentorial herniation and finally brainstem compression and death.

28. **D** Neither CT nor MRI were developed by 1957; CT was developed in 1971 in MRI in 1977, and while echocardiography was developed in 1953, it is not used in stroke diagnosis (Morrison, 2014).

29. **C** An uncommon, but serious complication of angiography is possible arterial tear, with bleeding into the retroperitoneal area. This would produce the symptoms of back pain and abdominal pain.

30. **A** Shellfish contain iodine, which is also present in most contrast dyes, making this allergy quite dangerous for contrast radiologic studies.

References

Alexander, S., Gallek, M., Presciutti, M., & Zrelak, P. (2012). Care of the patient with aneurysmal subarachnoid hemorrhage. AANN clinical practice guideline series. Retrieved from http://www.aann.org/pubs/content/guidelines.html

Connolly, E., Rabinstein, A., Carhuapoma, R., Derdeyn, C., Dion, J., Higashida, R. T., . . . Vespa, P. (2012). Guidelines for the management of aneurysmal subarachnoid hemorrhage: A guideline for healthcare professionals from the American Heart Association/American Stroke Association. *Stroke, 43,* 1711–1737.

Hemphill, J., Greenberg, S. M., Anderson, C. S., Becker, K., Bendok, B. R., Cushman M., . . . Woo, D. (2015). Guidelines for the management of spontaneous intracerebral hemorrhage: A guideline for healthcare professionals from the American Heart Association/American Stroke Association. *Stroke, 46,* 2032–2060.

Jauch, E., Saver, J., Adams, H., Bruno, A., Connors, J., Demaerschalk, B. M., . . . Yonas, H. (2013). Guidelines for the early management of patients with acute ischemic stroke: A guideline for healthcare professionals from the American Heart Association/American Stroke Association. *Stroke, 44,* 870–947.

Kernan, W. N., Ovbiagele, B., Black, H. R., Bravata, D. M., Chimowitz, M. I., Ezekowitz, M. D., . . . Wilson, J. A. (2014). Guidelines for the prevention of stroke in patients with stroke and transient ischemic attack: A guideline for healthcare professionals from the American Heart Association/American Stroke Association. *Stroke, 45,* 2160–2236.

Morrison, K. J. (2014). *Fast facts for stroke care nursing: An expert guide in a nutshell.* New York, NY: Springer Publishing.

Wijdicks, E. F. M., Sheth, K. N., Carter, B. S., Greer, D. M., Kasner, S. E., Kimberly, W. T., . . . Wintermark, M. (2014). Recommendations for the management of cerebral and cerebellar infarction and swelling: A statement for healthcare professionals from the American Heart Association/American Stroke Association. *Stroke, 45,* 1222–1238.

7

Acute Care

QUESTIONS

Neurologic Assessment

1. During National Institutes of Health Stroke Scale (NIHSS) scoring, your patient has intact sensation when each side is stimulated individually, but is unaware of being touched on the left side when both sides are stimulated simultaneously. What condition is apparent?

   A. Neuropathy
   B. Apraxia
   C. Extinction
   D. Paresthesia

2. Which is true of subarachnoid hemorrhage (SAH) scoring?

   A. The Hunt and Hess score is based on symptoms, and the Fisher scale score is based on amount/location of blood
   B. The Hunt and Hess score is based on amount/location of blood, and the Fisher scale score is based on symptoms
   C. The World Federation of Neurological Surgeons (WFNS) score is based on amount/location of blood on CT
   D. The WFNS score is based on age and symptoms

ANSWERS TO THIS SECTION CAN BE FOUND ON PAGE 91

3. The ABCD$_2$ score is used for which of the following situations?

   A. Calculating risk of vasospasm in subarachnoid hemorrhage (SAH)
   B. Determining eligibility for acute rehabilitation admission
   C. Predicting short-term risk of stroke in patients with transient ischemic attack (TIA)
   D. Calculating appropriate antithrombotic dose in nonvalvular atrial fibrillation

4. The neurologist completes a neurologic exam and tells you that the patient has the four Ds with crossed findings. Where is the patient's stroke?

   A. Tentorium
   B. Basal ganglia
   C. Midbrain
   D. Brainstem

5. Which of the following correctly represents the loss of half of the field of view on the same side in both eyes?

   A. Amaurosis fugax
   B. Bitemporal hemianopia
   C. Lateral hemianopia
   D. Homonymous hemianopia

6. When utilizing the Glasgow Coma Scale (GCS) to assess a stroke patient, which of the following is true?

   A. It is the most widely studied coma scale with high reliability in the stroke population
   B. Like the National Institutes of Health Stroke Scale (NIHSS), a low score is indicative of less deficit
   C. A normal motor score is possible for patients with hemiparesis
   D. Intubated patients are automatically scored a 2 for verbal response

7. Which cranial nerve (CN) is being assessed when you ask your patient to smile and raise his or her eyebrows?

   A. CN III
   B. CN VII
   C. CN I
   D. CN XII

8. Which cranial nerve (CN) is being assessed when you ask your patient to follow your finger with his or her eyes as you move it laterally/side to side?

    A. CN III
    B. CN II
    C. CN VI
    D. CN IV

9. In the National Institutes of Health Stroke Scale (NIHSS) score of a right middle cerebral artery (MCA) ischemic stroke patient, the patient scored 0 for motor arm bilaterally, 4 for motor leg on the left side, and was unable to perform the limb ataxia test successfully on the left leg. The patient was able to do it successfully on the right (unaffected) side. What total score does the patient get for limb ataxia?

    A. 2—Present in both upper and lower limbs
    B. 0—Absent
    C. 1—Present in upper *or* lower limb
    D. Calculating NIHSS score does not apply to this patient

10. The National Institutes of Health Stroke Scale (NIHSS) admission score has been proven valid as a predictor of discharge disposition. Which of the following is true of admission NIHSS scores?

    A. Score 1 to 5: anticipate discharge to home
    B. Score 6 to 13: anticipate discharge to acute rehabilitation facility
    C. Score higher than 13: anticipate discharge to extended care facility
    D. All of the above

11. A patient with a preadmission modified Rankin Scale (mRS) score of 1 was

    A. Independent in activities of daily living (ADL)
    B. Required some help, but was able to walk independently
    C. Required moderate assistance, and walked with walker
    D. Completely dependent for all ADL

12. Which is true of the Barthel Index (BI) score?

    A. It is a required functional score calculated daily by the bedside nurse
    B. The higher the score, the better the functional ability
    C. It has 100% correlative value with ischemic and hemorrhagic patients
    D. It is synonymous with FIM® score

13. Which of the following is a late finding in the neurologic assessment of a stroke patient?

    A. Headache
    B. Increased blood pressure (BP)
    C. Hippus response to light
    D. Decerebrate posturing

In the Intensive Care Unit

1. Patients with subarachnoid hemorrhage (SAH) should be monitored for which common complications of hemorrhagic stroke? Select all that are correct.

    A. Hyperactivity
    B. Hydrocephalus
    C. Cerebral vasospasm
    D. Seizure activity

2. Your patient just returned from having endovascular embolization of an arteriovenous malformation (AVM). Your nursing care for the next hour will include which of the following?

    A. Vital signs and neurologic checks q 15 minutes along with groin site checks
    B. Vital signs and neurologic checks q 15 minutes along with scalp incision checks
    C. Therapeutic hypothermia with goal of 35°C
    D. Education about the procedure and possible complications

3. Why is constipation prevented in the intensive care unit (ICU)?

    A. Neurologic ICU patients are prone to constipation secondary to cerebral edema
    B. Patients with constipation are more likely to develop Sundowner's syndrome
    C. Straining as a result of constipation causes blood pressure (BP) spikes
    D. Both A and B

4. Hypoxia in the intensive care unit (ICU) may be indicative of what condition?

    A. Aspiration pneumonia
    B. Hypoventilation

C. Airway obstruction

D. All of the above

5. Your intubated intracerebral hemorrhage patient is restless, despite sedation; the patient's blood pressure (BP) has risen to 176/90. What is your first action?

   A. Assess the patient for respiratory distress or other causes of pain

   B. Increase the dose of sedative within parameters and monitor for response

   C. Tell the patient care assistant (PCA) to notify the nurse who is going to cover for you while you go to lunch

   D. Document the change in your notes so that if further deterioration occurs, there will be clear trending of events

6. You are orienting a new intensive care unit (ICU) nurse who asks you why a 69-year-old ischemic stroke patient with no history of diabetes needs to have every 4 hours glucose checks. Your best response would be which of the following?

   A. "I have no idea either, but it's ordered, so we do it."

   B. "Hyperglycemia is common in ischemic stroke, even without a diabetes history, and can worsen outcomes if not controlled."

   C. "Hypoglycemia can occur suddenly after ischemic stroke as a result of increased intracranial pressure, and can worsen outcomes if not controlled."

   D. "Patients are known to deny a history of diabetes, so we test all our stroke patients."

7. Fever is common among stroke patients; what other complication should be anticipated for these patients as a result of fever?

   A. Urinary tract infection

   B. Aspiration pneumonia

   C. Cerebral edema

   D. Hypervolemia

8. While providing therapeutic cooling with an external cooling device, what condition will you be monitoring closely?

   A. Constipation

   B. Shivering

   C. Cognitive decline

   D. None of the above

9. In the report from the emergency department (ED) nurse, you are told that your stroke patient passed the swallow screen and took baby aspirin orally, along with a cup of decaf coffee. In what circumstance might the swallow screen be repeated during this patient's hospital stay?

   A. If there is no documentation of the swallow screen in the patient's medical record
   B. If there is a change in the National Institutes of Health Stroke Scale (NIHSS) score of 4 points or more, or clinical deterioration
   C. If the patient is noted to be drooling
   D. All of the above

10. You are caring for two ischemic stroke patients. Both had repeat imaging today. Patient A's was scheduled; patient B's was done as a result of new-onset headache and drowsiness. Both showed hemorrhagic transforma-tion. Which of the following would most likely be true?

    A. Patient A had petechial hemorrhage and patient B had parenchymal hemorrhage
    B. Patient A had parenchymal hemorrhage and patient B had petechial hemorrhage
    C. Both had intraventricular hemorrhage
    D. There is need for a second opinion on patient A's imaging as the patient was asymptomatic so could not have hemorrhagic transformation

11. What is the difference between cerebral salt wasting (CSW) and syn-drome of inappropriate antidiuretic hormone (SIADH)?

    A. There is no difference; CSW is the older term for SIADH
    B. CSW symptom is hyponatremia; SIADH symptom is hypernatremia
    C. CSW is often seen with subarachnoid hemorrhage (SAH) patients, and SIADH is often seen with ischemic stroke patients
    D. CSW is treated with sodium replacement and SIADH is treated with fluid restriction

12. Which of the following is *not* true about nursing care in the intensive care unit (ICU)?

    A. Postendovascular clot retrieval patients require monitoring of groin site
    B. Temperature monitoring is essential to facilitate treatment to main-tain normothermia

C. Systolic blood pressure (SBP) parameters for ischemic and intracerebral hemorrhage patients are 140 to 220 mmHg
D. Average patient load is one to two patients per nurse

13. Reperfusion syndrome is best described by which of the following?

A. Acute neurologic change after tissue plasminogen activator (tPA) infusion during second stroke event
B. Ipsilateral headache or contralateral neurologic deficit after successful clot retrieval
C. Acute onset hypotension following second pass of mechanical retrieval device
D. Ipsilateral seizure following successful embolization of aneurysm

14. What is the landmark for leveling an external ventricular drainage (EVD) catheter in a supine patient?

A. Tip of the nose
B. Clavicular notch
C. Tragus of the ear
D. Temporal window

15. A 58-year-old female patient was admitted yesterday with a small subarachnoid hemorrhage (SAH). Her medical history includes metabolic syndrome for which she was on a strict diet, having refused any other medical treatment. Her current vital signs are blood pressure (BP) 134/78, heart rate (HR) 86, respiratory rate (RR) 16, temperature 37°C, and pulse oxygen 88% on room air. What should be your next action?

A. Remove pulse oxygen sensor as she looks comfortable and vitals are stable
B. Recheck pulse oxygen and notify provider for oxygen order
C. Recheck pulse oxygen with next scheduled check of vital signs and neurologic status
D. Confirm that the patient is not feeling short of breath and document that

16. One of your patients is a married, 32-year-old mother of 10-year-old twins. She suffered a hemorrhagic stroke a week ago, and things are looking grim. The patient's sister refuses to accept the fact that she may

not survive; her husband is saying that she would not have wanted to live this way, and is frankly talking about whether he should discontinue support. What is your role as a bedside nurse?

    A. Avoid the topic each time either of them mentions it, as it is up to the social worker to deal with this

    B. Communicate the situation to the health care team and participate in a family meeting

    C. Sit the sister down and get her to understand how unlikely recovery is

    D. None of the above

17. Most deaths following middle cerebral artery (MCA) occlusion in older patients occur during what time period?

    A. During the first 24 hours

    B. 3 to 4 days

    C. 7 to 10 days

    D. 30 to 60 days

18. Mr. Poole, your patient in Room 408, is proving to be quite challenging to keep in bed. He is impulsive and does not seem to be aware of one side of his body. In what area did his stroke occur?

    A. Left cerebellum

    B. Right basal ganglia

    C. Right parietal lobe

    D. Left temporal lobe

In the Stroke Unit

1. On Day 7 postcoiling, your aneurysmal subarachnoid hemorrhage (SAH) patient says she feels good enough to go home and wonders why the doctor said she has to stay another 3 to 4 days. Your answer would be which of the following?

    A. Her stroke education has not been completed yet

    B. She is at high risk of rebleed

    C. She is at high risk of vasospasm

    D. Her anticoagulant has not yet reached therapeutic level

2. Your patient with left hemisphere stroke complains of right arm pain and scores it as 3 of 10 on the pain scale. What would your next nursing action be?

   A. Educate the patient that pain is a good sign that sensation is intact
   B. Notify the provider and anticipate repeat CT scan
   C. Document as new pain and include in report to next shift
   D. Reposition the patient, ensuring that the affected arm is well supported

3. Your new patient complains of headache and you have an order for acetaminophen PO. You are about to administer a dose when you remember that you were not told whether the patient had a dysphagia screen done in the emergency department (ED). Your next step is to

   A. Give the medication anyway because the patient seems alert and able to swallow okay
   B. Call the ED and leave a message for the nurse to call you back with the answer
   C. Perform the dysphagia screen now
   D. Apologize and explain that you will be back in a few minutes after you check the patient's chart

4. On rounds, Dr. Hamilton, the stroke neurologist, is reviewing Mrs. Smith's medical record. It is Day 2 for this 72-year-old with a lacunar stroke. What would have made the provider quiz the patient about family history of diabetes?

   A. Hgb A1C of 9%
   B. Fasting glucose of 122
   C. Small vessel disease on CT
   D. Remembering another current patient—same last name—with diabetes

5. During rounds, your stroke patient begs Dr. Harms to let him have water, despite the thorough explanation you provided to the patient earlier that he failed the bedside swallow screen and the speech and language pathologist (SLP) will need to do a more thorough evaluation before he can have anything to drink. Dr. Harms states that as this patient can speak clearly and is alert, he must be able to swallow

adequately. The provider orders the patient to have liquids as desired. Your best response would be to:

A. Repeat the evidence-based dysphagia screen
B. Accept that the provider is a doctor and in charge, so you get the patient some ice water
C. Ignore the provider's order, and refuse to give the patient water
D. Page the SLP stat to come and evaluate the patient

6. Postural (orthostatic) hypotension is considered when which of the following conditions is present?

A. A 10-mmHg drop in systolic blood pressure (SBP) after 2 hours of sitting out of bed in a chair
B. A 20-mmHg drop in SBP within 5 minutes of standing after supine rest
C. Hemorrhagic stroke—postural hypotension is not applicable to ischemic stroke
D. A 20-mmHg drop in SBP after initiation of new antihypertensive medication

7. Which of the following is *not* a recommended treatment for prevention of venous thrombosis?

A. Low–molecular weight heparin
B. Elastic compression stockings, also called thromboembolic disease (TED) stockings
C. Intermittent pneumatic compression (IPC) devices, also called sequential compression devices (SCD)
D. Heparinoids

8. For which of the following conditions would you be most concerned about complications with use of anticoagulation for deep vein thrombosis (DVT) prophylaxis?

A. Anterior cerebral artery ischemic stroke
B. Secured aneurysmal subarachnoid hemorrhage (SAH)
C. Basal ganglia ischemic stroke
D. Subcortical intracerebral hemorrhage (ICH)

9. Which nursing measure would best reduce the risk of urinary tract infection (UTI) poststroke?

   A. Encouragement of oral fluid intake
   B. Regular schedule of bladder elimination
   C. Administration of as-needed acetaminophen
   D. Close monitoring of intake and output

10. Why are stroke patients at higher risk for urinary tract infection (UTI)?

    A. High incidence of urinary incontinence and retention due to neurologic insult
    B. Poor hygiene associated with hemiparesis results in increased risk
    C. Intolerance of prophylactic antibiotics increases risk
    D. Inadequate bladder catheter care by neuroscience staff increases risk

11. Nursing care for stroke patients includes ensuring that they are repositioned frequently. The reason that this is more critical for stroke patients than for other patients is that

    A. In addition to neurologic damage with an infarct, there is also dermatologic damage resulting in increased susceptibility to skin breakdown
    B. There are regulatory requirements for reporting skin breakdown related to stroke that significantly impact reimbursements
    C. Due to motor and sensory deficits, stroke patients often cannot reposition themselves off pressure points or feel the pain associated with early skin breakdown
    D. Repositioning of stroke patients is not a nursing care priority

12. In the report, you are told that Mr. Todd, a 58-year-old with a right middle cerebral artery (MCA) stroke is experiencing neglect. How will you incorporate this information into your nursing plan of care?

    A. Turn bed around so that the patient's left side is facing the door
    B. Approach Mr. Todd from the right side
    C. Place a sign over the bed indicating that all activities are to be initiated from the left side
    D. Place the bedside table on the left side

13. Your patient's neurologist documented that the patient had a crypto-genic stroke. You are unfamiliar with this term and look it up. Which of the following is true about what you learned?

    A. The patient has a familial tendency toward stroke from a distant relative
    B. The likelihood of death within 1 year is 80%
    C. The cause of the stroke is unknown despite a full workup
    D. The patient had no symptoms prior to the stroke

14. Which of the following examples illustrates aphasia?

    A. A patient who refers to a fork as a ring, and a call bell as a muffin
    B. A patient whose speech is slurred and unintelligible
    C. A patient who cannot initiate a sentence, but can repeat correctly after you
    D. A patient who refuses to speak

15. Your ischemic patient had mechanical thrombectomy. The report states that the patient was recanalized. You know that this means

    A. A second circulatory path was able to be established
    B. Blood flow was restored to the arterial occlusion site
    C. Their groin site was closed with the plug-style device
    D. Both groins were punctured so assessment of both sites is essential

16. Your ischemic patient was admitted from the emergency department (ED) to the stroke unit at 10:00 p.m. yesterday (Thursday), after receiving IV tissue plasminogen activator (tPA) at 9:00 p.m. It is now Friday at 9:00 p.m. and you know that for your patient to have the best outcome according to evidence-based guidelines, you need to accomplish which of the following?

    A. Documentation of vital signs and neurologic checks every 15 minutes until midnight
    B. Risk factor education prior to midnight
    C. Documentation of dysphagia screen prior to each medication administration
    D. Administration of aspirin between 9:00 p.m. and midnight

17. You recently attended the International Stroke Conference (ISC) and learned about the different levels and classes of evidence and what they mean. You are preparing to do an in service for your colleagues. Which of the following is correct information to include?

    A. "Level" refers to the estimate of certainty based on size of population studied, and "class" refers to the estimate of benefit versus risk
    B. Class I, Level A recommendations have the highest likelihood of benefit
    C. Both A and B are correct
    D. The terms "level" and "class" both refer to the degree of expertise of the investigators

18. You receive a 50-year-old ischemic stroke patient from the neurologic intensive care unit (ICU) who is in a wheelchair and wearing a helmet. You know that the patient will wear the helmet at all times except for which situation?

    A. During daily hygiene
    B. During occupational therapy
    C. During visiting hours
    D. At meal times

19. Your 80-year-old patient and his family have just elected for do not resuscitate (DNR) status due to his diagnosis 6 months ago of metastatic lung cancer and now this ischemic stroke. Which of the following describes the changes to his care?

    A. Cessation of daily lab work
    B. Reduction of frequency of vital signs and neurologic checks to once daily
    C. Cessation of therapy services
    D. None of the above

20. Right before lunch, the patient care assistant mentions that a patient coughed a lot while being fed breakfast. Your best next action would be which of the following?

    A. Monitor the patient's temperature and breath sounds for the next 24 hours
    B. Repeat the swallow screen right away before any more medications or lunch

C. Ask the patient if there are any other symptoms of a cold

D. Remind the patient care assistant to have the patient tuck the chin with each swallow

21. Your stroke patient's monitor shows atrial fibrillation. She says she feels fine and does not mind that rhythm so does not want any procedures to treat it, and does not like blood thinners. What is your best response?

A. Explain that untreated atrial fibrillation results in extreme fatigue that inhibits rehabilitation

B. Explain that untreated atrial fibrillation can deteriorate to ventricular fibrillation

C. Explain that untreated atrial fibrillation puts the patient at risk for another stroke, and is likely the cause of this stroke

D. Accept the patient's right to choose the treatment plan and document that choice

22. In reviewing your patient's medical history, you note a risk factor for ischemic stroke. Which of the following did you see?

A. Factor V Leiden

B. Thrombocytopenia

C. Elevated creatinine

D. Hypokalemia

23. In providing education to your transient ischemic attack (TIA) patient, which of the statements by the patient indicates that an understanding of the information?

A. "TIAs are usually caused by small bleeds in the brain that resolve on their own."

B. "It is important to call 911 immediately if I experience these symptoms again because it could mean that I am having a stroke."

C. "Because TIAs don't cause permanent damage, I do not need to worry if I have another one."

D. "TIAs are usually caused by brief synaptic gaps in the brain during extreme physical activity."

24. The provider is reviewing the international normalized ratio (INR) results of a patient with a history of embolic stroke who is now on warfarin. Which of the following indicates a therapeutic value for this patient?

A. 1.4
B. 4.5
C. 2.5
D. 0.5

25. A 61-year-old female subarachnoid hemorrhagic patient is getting ready to be discharged to home. As you are reviewing instructions with her son for what to do if she develops stroke symptoms, which response indicates that he needs more teaching?

    A. "I should take her to the emergency room right away."
    B. "I should note the time that the symptoms started."
    C. "I should call 911 right away."
    D. "I should make sure that I have her medication list."

26. Which of the following would be included in the discharge education of an ischemic stroke patient going home?

    A. Make every effort to keep all follow-up appointments scheduled.
    B. Eat a diet low in saturated fat and high in sodium
    C. Both A and B
    D. Neither A nor B

27. Your stroke patient has been found to have 85% right carotid stenosis and is scheduled for carotid endarterectomy tomorrow. Your patient asks if vision will return to normal postop. What is your best response?

    A. Removal of the plaque sometimes results in reversal of symptoms
    B. Carotid endarterectomy is for prevention of another stroke; it will not change the damage done already from a stroke
    C. The patient will receive extensive vision therapy after surgery that will restore vision
    D. Excuse yourself and notify the provider that the patient is not back to baseline, so surgery will need to be delayed

28. It is Day 3 for your left middle cerebral artery (MCA) stroke patient. You observe the patient care assistant working with the patient. For which of the following would you need to intervene?

    A. The patient care assistant assists the patient to ambulate to the bathroom and back to bed

B. The patient care assistant assists the patient with a bath

C. The patient care assistant sets up the patient's lunch tray and leaves the room

D. The patient care assistant places the blood pressure cuff on the left arm

29. A small patent foramen ovale (PFO) is discovered on an ischemic stroke patient's echocardiography. Minimal right to left shunting is seen with the Valsalva maneuver. Which of the following is the most appropriate treatment for this patient?

A. Aspirin 325 mg/day

B. Warfarin with a target international normalized ratio (INR) of 1.5 to 2.5

C. Warfarin with a target INR of 1.5 to 2.5 and aspirin 81 mg/day

D. Warfarin with a target INR of 1.5 to 2.5 and referral for PFO closure

7

Acute Care

ANSWERS

Neurologic Assessment

1. **C** Extinction is the result of parietal lobe damage and is characterized by the inability to discern stimulation on the side contralateral to the infarct when stimulated on both sides simultaneously. With extinction, sensation is intact when each side is individually stimulated—only lost with double, or multiple, stimuli simultaneously. Neuropathy is a condition of peripheral nerves, usually in the lower extremities, characterized by numbness, tingling, and pain. Paresthesia is also a peripheral nerve condition characterized by numbness, tingling, and a pins-and-needles sensation.

2. **A** Hunt and Hess, Fisher scale, and WFNS scores are all used in SAH patients, but Hunt and Hess is based on what symptoms are present, and Fisher is based on the amount of blood present, while the WFNS is based on the Glasgow Coma Scale score and presence or absence of motor deficit (Morrison, 2014).

3. **C** The $ABCD_2$ score predicts short-term risk of stroke in patients with TIA. The acronym stands for age, blood pressure, clinical features, duration of symptoms, and diabetes (Morrison, 2014).

4. **D** Classic in brainstem strokes, the four Ds are dysphagia, dysarthria, diplopia, and dysmetria, and crossed signs indicate that motor and sensory deficits do not match the classic pattern seen in hemispheric strokes.

5. **D** Homonymous hemianopia is the loss of half of the field of view on the same side in both eyes. It is also referred to as a homonymous hemianopsia. It occurs because of the way part of the optic nerve fibers from each eye crossover as they pass to the back of the brain. The visual images that we see on the right side travel from both eyes to the left side of the brain, while the visual images we see on the left side in each eye travels to the right side of the brain. Therefore, damage to the right side of the posterior portion of the brain can cause a loss of the left field of view in both eyes. Likewise, damage to the left posterior brain can cause a loss of the right field of vision (Windsor & Windsor, 2004).

6. **C** The Glasgow Coma Scale was developed in 1974 to evaluate the depth of decreased consciousness and coma in the head injury population. The range of score is 0 to 15, with points deducted for deficit, so the higher the score, the better the patient status. The motor component only tests for best effort, so a stroke patient with hemiparesis could still get a normal motor score owing to being able to demonstrate motor strength with the unaffected limb. Therefore it does not have high reliability with the stroke population.

7. **B** CN VII, the facial nerve, is involved in smiling and raising eyebrows; CN III, the oculomotor nerve, is involved in eye movements; CN I, the olfactory nerve, is involved in smell; and CN XII, the hypoglossal nerve, is involved in tongue movement.

8. **A** CN III, the oculomotor nerve, is involved in eye movements; CN II, the optic nerve, is involved in vision or visual confrontation; CN VI, the Abducens nerve, is involved in lateral vision; and CN IV, the Trochlear nerve, is involved in looking down toward the floor.

9. **B** The rules for scoring ataxia in the NIHSS state that you should only score an inability as ataxia if the inability to perform the task is out of proportion to the patient's weakness. Since this patient scored a 4 for motor ability on the left leg, the patient has no movement at all. This patient's inability to do the ataxia exam is due to weakness, not to inability to coordinate the movement, so does not get an ataxia score.

10. **D** Research evidence has proven the admission NIHSS to be a reliable predictor of discharge disposition based on the ranges described in the question.

11. **A** The mRS is a commonly used scale for measuring the degree of disability or dependence in the daily activities of the stroke population. The scores range from 0 to 6, with 0 being no deficits, and 6 being dead. A score of 1 is defined as no significant disability, able to carry out all usual activities, despite some symptoms. A score of 2 to 5 indicates varying degrees of dependence.

12. **B** The Barthel Index is used to measure performance in specific activities of daily living (ADL). The 10 areas are scored 1 to 10, with a total score possible of 100. The higher the score, the more likely the patient is to be independent. It is not a required daily score for stroke-certified centers, and it is not as highly correlated with hemorrhagic stroke as with ischemic stroke. It is not synonymous with FIM, which is Functional Independence Measure, a scale used in the postacute rehabilitation setting.

13. **D** Decerebrate posturing is characterized by a rigid, possibly arched, spine, rigidly extended arms and legs, and plantar flexion. It is seen in the stroke population in patients with increased intracranial pressure to the point of pressure on the brainstem, or herniation. Headache, increased blood pressure, and pupil changes occur earlier in the setting of acute stroke.

In the Intensive Care Unit

1. **B, C, D** Hydrocephalus develops when the blood clots over the arachnoid villi, blocking flow of cerebrospinal fluid; vasospasm develops because the blood is irritating the outer layer of the arteries causing them to spasm; and seizure activity is the result of the irritation of the blood on the surrounding tissue—think of it as a short circuit of the brain's electrical system.

2. **A** Endovascular embolization is done via an arterial approach, not transcranial, so groin checks would be done along with the every 15 minutes vitals and neurologic checks.

3. **C** Straining involves the Valsalva maneuver, which results in transient high blood pressure. For patients with new stroke, and possibly

inactive autoregulation, blood pressure spikes could be dangerous. Autoregulation is present in normal, healthy brains. It is the mechanism that keeps a steady intracerebral pressure, regardless of what is going on in the body. When the brain is injured, autoregulation may be temporarily inactivated, so the brain is particularly susceptible to highs and lows of systemic blood pressure.

4. **D** Hypoxia could result from all three: aspiration pneumonia because the inflammatory process produces excess mucus and secretions that inhibit oxygen absorption and exchange; hypoventilation because inadequate inflation or low respiratory rate limits the amount of oxygen exchanged; and airway obstruction because if oxygenated air cannot get into the lungs, it cannot get absorbed into the blood.

5. **A** If your restless patient is unable to communicate what is wrong, assessment of possible causes of distress, respiratory or pain, will help to determine the appropriate treatment. Just increasing the dose of sedative is dangerous because if the cause of the restlessness is found and resolved, there is risk of oversedation and hypotension, which is not good for the patient's injured brain.

6. **B** Research has shown that sustained hyperglycemia after stroke is associated with worse outcomes, even in patients without diabetes.

7. **C** Fever results in cerebral edema owing to the breakdown of the blood–brain barrier.

8. **B** Shivering is a common challenge with surface cooling, and if not controlled can raise the body temperature negating the impact of the cooling therapy.

9. **D** Even though you were told in the report that the patient passed a swallow screen, if it is not documented the most prudent thing is to simply repeat it, as it is not a difficult process. For a patient with a change in neurologic status or an NIHSS increase of 4 points or more, you should anticipate that the ability to swallow safely may also have changed; and for a patient who had been deemed safe to swallow but is drooling, repeating the swallow screen is essential, as new drooling is closely linked to swallow ability.

10. *A* Petechial hemorrhage is defined as patchy hemorrhage, and patients are usually asymptomatic; parenchymal hemorrhage is defined as hemorrhage with mass effect, and patients are usually symptomatic (Morrison, 2014, p. 125).

11. *D* CSW and SIADH are not synonymous; CSW is caused by excessive removal of salt by the kidneys and is treated with sodium replacement; SIADH is dilutional low sodium and is treated with fluid restriction (Morrison, 2014, p. 124).

12. *C* The blood pressure parameters for ischemic and hemorrhagic patients are not the same, with hemorrhagic patients having a lower range of acceptable blood pressure than ischemic patients.

13. *B* Reperfusion syndrome is described as the inflammatory reaction to the restoration of blood flow to an ischemic area with common symptoms being ipsilateral headache and contralateral neurologic deficits. It is associated with postprocedure hypertension and treatment is tight management of the blood pressure. It is not a second stroke event, although without good medical management, that could occur. It also would not result from an aneurysm embolization as that does not result in restored circulation to an ischemic area.

14. *C* The external landmark for leveling an EVD is the tragus of the ear; the internal landmark is the foramen of Monroe.

15. *B* Even though the patient does not appear to be in respiratory distress, the injured brain needs better oxygenation than an 88% saturation provides, so notify the provider if that is what it is on recheck.

16. *B* The best response in this situation is to make sure the health care team is aware, and that there is a family meeting in which as many members of the team as possible participate.

17. *B* Most deaths from large MCA infarcts occur in the first week but usually not during the first day. At that time, the infarct may still be evolving. The cause of death is cerebral edema, which is not yet full blown on the first day.

18. *C* Right parietal lobe infarcts are associated with impulsivity and extinction, or neglect of the left side. Cerebellar strokes are associated with lack

of coordination (ataxia) and imbalance; basal ganglia strokes are associated with lacunar strokes that are pure sensory or pure motor; temporal lobe strokes are associated with receptive language problems and memory deficit.

In the Stroke Unit

1. **C** The risk of vasospasm is highest in the first 10 days after SAH; the risk of rebleed is highest in the first 24 hours after SAH. If the patient had been on anticoagulation therapy and was having it resumed, it would been restarted safely earlier than Day 7, so an additional 3 to 4 days as stated by the doctor would not make sense.

2. **D** Patients with hemiparesis of the upper extremity can experience arm pain as a result of poor technique used by staff when repositioning or mobilizing them. It can also result from the weight of the arm pulling down if unsupported. The best next action would be to reposition and ensure that the arm is properly supported and assess for possible relief of pain.

3. **C** Most dysphagia screens are simple to do, so the best action would be to go ahead and do a brief screen so that the patient can receive the pain medication as quickly and safely as possible.

4. **A** Hemoglobin A1C is an indicator of the average level of blood sugar over the past 2 to 3 months. A level greater than 6.5% meets the threshold for diagnosis of diabetes; a fasting blood sugar greater than 126 also meets the threshold.

5. **D** Paging the SLP stat would be best to ensure the patient receives the appropriate evaluation as soon as possible. As you had just performed the swallow screen shortly before rounds, there is no need to repeat it, but there is actually no harm either, so answer A would be okay.

6. **B** Postural hypotension is defined as occurring within 5 minutes of standing from supine. The term has become more broadly used for patients whose BP drops as a result of sitting for an extended period, but it is technically not postural hypotension (Arbique, Cheek, Welliver, & Vongpatanasin, 2014).

7. **B** With TED stockings, the benefit does not outweigh the risk of harm. In the acute population, there is a high likelihood of the stockings being applied by someone other than the patient, and with possible language or sensory deficits, the patient cannot always communicate, or be aware, if there is poor fit and compromised circulation or skin integrity (Dennis et al., 2009).

8. **D** Anticoagulation during the acute phase of stroke recovery is most risky in ICH, unsecured aneurysms, and large territory ischemic stroke patients.

9. **B** Facilitation of regular bladder emptying limits the risk of UTI because of less retention time.

10. **A** Patients with neurologic injury, such as stroke, are at risk for incontinence and retention. Retention of urine in the bladder is a risk for UTI.

11. **C** Stroke patients with hemiparesis have limited ability to reposition themselves; stroke patients with sensory deficit are not aware of the warning signs of pain that most people feel when pressure points are developing (Alexander, 2013).

12. **B** A patient with a right-sided infarct who experiences neglect will not be aware of the left side, so initial approach, and the bedside table, should be on the right side.

13. **C** Cryptogenic stroke is defined as a stroke that has no definite cause, all known causes have been ruled out. *Cryptic* means mysterious, so it makes sense that cryptogenic means without known cause.

14. **A** Aphasia is a term that refers to many types of language dysfunction, and inaccurate naming is one of them. Slurred speech would be dysarthria; inability to initiate would be apraxia; refusal to speak would be stubbornness.

15. **B** Recanalization is defined as restoration of a lumen in a blood vessel following thrombotic occlusion, or reopening of a blocked vessel.

16. **D** Evidence has shown that early antithrombotic administration leads to better patient outcomes. Stroke performance measure 5 (STK 5) requires the antithrombotic to be administered by end of Day 2 (midnight). What

makes this case challenging is that the patient got tPA, and you cannot administer it for 24 hours post tPA (so not before 9:00 p.m.), leaving only a few hours to give it within the best practice parameters.

17. **C** The system for determining the levels and classes of evidence in making clinical care decisions was developed in 1979 through a collaborative process among physicians, scientists, and researchers. "Level" refers to the estimate of certainty based on size of population studied, and "class" refers to the estimate of benefit versus risk; there are four classes, and three levels utilized, and a Class I, Level A is the highest level of recommendation. The table showing all the levels and classes can be found in most of the American Heart Association/American Stroke Association Guidelines (Burns, Rohrich, & Chung, 2011).

18. **A** Some stroke patients (usually younger patients with large territory strokes) have a hemicraniectomy performed to allow for brain swelling and to prevent herniation or secondary stroke from compression. Without the bone flap (piece of bone), they are at risk of brain injury so they wear a helmet at all times, except for during daily hygiene.

19. **D** A DNR order simply means that if the patient were to experience cardiac or respiratory arrest, there would be no cardiopulmonary resuscitation (CPR) or intubation. It does not mean that care stops or changes in any other way.

20. **B** Coughing is a sign of possible swallowing difficulty, and the patient should be rescreened right away, so that no more medications or food are given without determination of swallowing ability. You will also monitor temperature and breath sounds, but the most important thing to do right away is to rescreen.

21. **C** While patients have a right to make treatment decisions, that is only after they have received the proper education and information. Make sure the patient understands the consequence of an untreated atrial fibrillation, which is another stroke.

22. **A** Factor V Leiden is a mutation of one of the clotting factors in the blood called Factor V, which can increase the chance of developing blood clots (thrombophilia).

23. *B* TIAs are a classic warning sign that a stroke might occur in the future; TIA is to stroke like angina is to myocardial infarction. Patients who understand this would know that if they have symptoms again, they will call 911.

24. *C* An INR of 2.5 is within therapeutic range for most anticoagulated patients, 2.5 to 3.5.

25. *A* Evidence has shown that patients who arrive via emergency medical services (EMS) have faster access to identification and treatment of their stroke, so the son stating that he would take her to the emergency department (ED) indicates the need for more education about the importance of calling 911.

26. *A* The only correct answer is the importance of keeping follow-up appointments; B is incorrect because it says high-sodium diet, which is just the opposite of what is correct.

27. *B* It is important to control expectations, and carotid endarterectomy is a prevention measure—it will not change the fact that the patient has had a stroke resulting in vision change. The patient may be getting vision therapy, but it is not correct to say that it will restore the vision, as there are no guarantees that this will happen.

28. *C* MCA territory strokes usually involve sizable brain tissue being affected, which usually is accompanied by cerebral edema. On Day 3, the patient will likely still be groggy, and should not be left alone to feed himself or herself.

29. *A* A multicenter study comparing aspirin and warfarin for treatment of stroke patients with PFO found no difference in stroke risk between treatment groups but found a significantly higher rate of hemorrhage in the warfarin-treated group. PFO closure would not be recommended in a patient with a first stroke who has not yet been treated with an antithrombotic medication.

References

Alexander, S. (Ed.). (2013). *Evidence-based nursing care for stroke and neurovascular conditions.* Ames, IA: Wiley-Blackwell.

Arbique, D., Cheek, D., Welliver, M., & Vongpatanasin, W. (2014). Management of neurogenic orthostatic hypotension. *Journal of the American Medical Directors Association, 15*(4), 234–239.

Burns, P. B., Rohrich, R. J., & Chung, K. C. (2011). The levels of evidence and their role in evidence-based medicine. Retrieved from https://www.ncbi.nlm.nih.gov/pmc/articles/PMC3124652

Dennis, M., Sandercock, P. A. G., Reid, J., Graham, C., Murray, G., Venables, G., . . . Bowler, G. (2009). Effectiveness of thigh-length graduated compression stockings to reduce the risk of deep vein thrombosis after stroke (CLOTS trial 1): A multicentre, randomised controlled trial. *The Lancet, 373*(9679), 1958–1965.

Morrison, K. J. (2014). *Fast facts for stroke care nursing: An expert guide in a nutshell.* New York, NY: Springer Publishing.

Windsor, L., & Windsor, R. (2004). Hemianopsia (hemianopia). Retrieved from http://www.hemianopsia.net

8

Medications

QUESTIONS

1. Of the following antiplatelet agents, one is indicated for primary prevention, while others are indicated for secondary prevention. Which is the primary prevention agent?

    A. Dipyridamole/aspirin (Aggrenox)
    B. Aspirin
    C. Clopidogrel (Plavix)
    D. Ticlopidine (Ticlid)

2. The term "antiplatelet" agent is used because the mechanism of action is to

    A. Increase platelet resistance of the blood–brain barrier
    B. Inhibit platelet production in the liver
    C. Decrease platelet passage through the cell membrane
    D. Decrease platelet aggregation in the bloodstream

3. Your patient with atrial fibrillation has just been started on warfarin. What will be part of your medication education for them?

    A. Eliminate salads and foods rich in vitamin K
    B. Intake of salads and foods rich in vitamin K should be consistent

ANSWERS TO THIS SECTION CAN BE FOUND ON PAGE 108

    C. Never take medication on an empty stomach

    D. Avoid physical activity to limit bruising risk

4. Your patient has just had a nasogastric (NG) tube inserted for enteral feeding. You have received confirmation of correct placement in the stomach, and initiated feeding 2 hours ago. Which of the following is now safe to administer via this route?

    A. Rivaroxaban (Xarelto)

    B. Dabigatran (Pradaxa)

    C. Apixaban (Eliquis)

    D. Abciximab (ReoPro)

5. Which of the statements below best describes the action of alteplase?

    A. Promotes fibrinolysis of fibrin clots

    B. Directly inhibits free and fibrin-bound thrombin

    C. Directly inhibits free and clot-bound factor Xa

    D. Inhibits activation of vitamin K–dependent clotting factors

6. In the emergency department (ED), alteplase has been ordered for Mr. Paine. The following is the patient's home medication list. Which of the medications would make you more alert for orolingual angioedema?

    A. Metformin

    B. Simvastatin

    C. Lisinopril

    D. Aspirin

7. For Mr. Paine, which of these home medications might be responsible for his dry, nonproductive cough?

    A. Metformin (Glucophage)

    B. Simvastatin (Zocor)

    C. Lisinopril (Prinivil, Zestril)

    D. Aspirin

8. Which of these lipid-lowering agents has the best primary and secondary risk reduction?

    A. Atorvastatin (Lipitor)

    B. Gemfibrozil (Lopid)

C. Fenofibrate (Tricor)

D. Niacin

9. Your patient has been ordered to receive 23.4% saline, 30 mL, over 20 minutes. What do you tell the patient and the family about this treatment?

A. The patient will need to be transferred to the long-term acute care (LTAC) unit in order for insurance to cover this therapy

B. Reducing blood viscosity reduces risk of seizure

C. Saline is equivalent to blood viscosity and it helps to hydrate

D. Concentrated saline helps to reduce brain swelling

10. For which of the lipid-lowering agents would you include education about a possible side effect of flushing?

A. Atorvastatin (Lipitor)

B. Niacin

C. Cholestyramine (Questran)

D. Simvastatin (Zocor)

11. Your patient's list of home medications includes a long-acting insulin. Which of the following would that be?

A. Insulin lispro (Humalog)

B. Insulin aspart (NovoLog)

C. Insulin glargine (Lantus)

D. Insulin glulisine (Apidra)

12. Your patient just returned from having a CT angiogram. You might have an order to hold which of the following medications for 48 hours?

A. Simvastatin (Zocor)

B. Metformin (Glucophage)

C. Aspirin

D. Cardizem (Diltiazem)

13. During the morning assessment, Mr. Smith tells you that he does not think recovery will be sufficient to make him want to keep living. What is your responsibility? Choose all that apply.

A. Reassure Mr. Smith that his feelings are not unusual, and that he will have help to deal with these feelings

B. Report this conversation to the provider

C. Realize that stroke patients often say things like this and it is best to let it pass quietly to avoid embarrassing them

D. Monitor Mr. Smith's mood and behavior for further changes

14. Which medication do you anticipate to be ordered for a patient with signs of depression?
   A. Escitalopram (Lexapro)
   B. Paroxetine (Paxil)
   C. Sertraline (Zoloft)
   D. Any of the above

15. When you bring the first dose of antidepressant to your patient, and she says she does not want to take "crazy people pills," what is your best response?
   A. Antidepressants may enhance neurogenesis and thus functional recovery
   B. Antidepressants facilitate pain management and will make therapy less painful
   C. Antidepressants inhibit appetite which may result in weight loss
   D. If you do not take this medication, your doctor will be angry

16. Your 20-year-old right–middle cerebral artery (MCA) territory stroke patient is awake and complaining of left shoulder pain. He has a history of a severe back injury from a snow boarding accident last year. He asks for his lollipop. What is he referring to?
   A. Fentanyl buccal route
   B. Dilaudid oral solution frozen
   C. Oxycontin oral solution frozen
   D. MS Contin buccal route

17. Which antipyretic could be given to your febrile, postoperative patient without concern for antiplatelet effect?
   A. Ibuprofen (Advil, Motrin)
   B. Aspirin
   C. Acetaminophen (Tylenol)
   D. None, they all impact platelet aggregation

18. Which of the following medications dissolves blood clots?
    A. Warfarin (Coumadin)
    B. Alteplase (Activase)
    C. IV heparin
    D. Rivaroxaban (Xarelto)

19. Your emergency department (ED) patient has arrived at 2 hours 30 minutes from symptom onset and Dr. Jones says to get the IV alteplase ready stat. The patient's weight is 250 lbs. How much of the dose will be given as a bolus?
    A. 10 mg
    B. 14 mg
    C. 9 mg
    D. 20 mg

20. In the sign-off report at 7 p.m., the nurse tells you that the patient arrived at 2 p.m. to the stroke unit with a diagnosis of middle cerebral artery (MCA) stroke. Aspirin 81 mg orally was ordered, but was held owing to the patient failing the dysphagia screen. How do you respond?
    A. Antithrombotics are to be administered by end of hospital day 2 or the length of stay will be extended
    B. Antithrombotics need to be given early for best patient outcomes, so you will get an order for suppository right away
    C. Antithrombotics are really only important in lacunar strokes, so a delay is not a problem
    D. If this patient got alteplase, antithrombotics need to be given within 24 hours of alteplase dose

21. In the emergency department (ED), a patient became somnolent after complaining of a headache. After reviewing the CT and labs (intracerebral hemorrhage and international normalized ratio [INR] 2.5), the provider orders stat fresh frozen plasma (FFP). Which oral anticoagulant was the patient taking prior to admission?
    A. Apixaban (Eliquis)
    B. Dabigatran (Pradaxa)
    C. Rivaroxaban (Xarelto)
    D. Warfarin (Coumadin)

22. In the stroke clinic, Mr. Small and his wife are arguing when you enter
the room. He has recently been started on warfarin and they cannot agree
about whether it is important to mention the following item. When you
hear what it is, you tell them that it is important.
    A. He started taking gingko for memory help
    B. He has developed an appetite for peaches
    C. He is regaining sensation in his left thumb
    D. He has been having unusual dreams about cats

23. Headache occurs in up to 40% of patients taking which medication?
    A. Dipyridamole/aspirin (Aggrenox)
    B. Metoprolol (Lopressor)
    C. Rivaroxaban (Xarelto)
    D. Nicardipine (Cardene)

24. The neuroscience ICU nurse notified the intensivist team that the patient
just had three seizures, each of 50 seconds' duration. Which medication
is the first-line agent for this situation?
    A. Levetiracetam (Keppra)
    B. Valproic acid (Depakote)
    C. Lorazepam (Ativan)
    D. Pentobarbital (Nembutal)

25. How often should patients with insulin drips have their blood glucose
checked?
    A. Every 3 to 6 hours
    B. Every 2 to 4 hours
    C. Every 1 to 2 hours
    D. Every other day

26. Which is true of the U.S. Food and Drug Administration's (FDA) approval
of alteplase (Activase)?
    A. It was based on the National Institute of Neurological Disorders and
    Stroke (NINDS) recombinant tissue plasminogen activator (rt-PA)
    Stroke Trial of 1995
    B. It was approved despite a 12% intracerebral hemorrhage rate
    C. It was approved for 3 to 4.5 hours from onset in select populations
    D. It was approved for 3 hours from onset

27. The appropriate administration of alteplase includes which of the following?
    A. It should be given with an 18-gauge or larger needle
    B. 10% is given as a bolus over 1 minute
    C. Shaking the vial vigorously enhances the dissolution of the powder
    D. If anaphylaxis is suspected, the rate should be reduced by 50% and the provider notified

28. Which medication is Class I, Level of Evidence A for use in aneurysmal subarachnoid hemorrhage?
    A. IV magnesium sulfate
    B. Oral nimodipine
    C. Oral papaverine
    D. Oral amlodipine

29. On what schedule will a patient who receives alteplase have vital signs and neurologic checks monitored?
    A. Every 15 minutes for 2 hours, then every 30 minutes for 6 hours, then hourly for 16 hours
    B. Every 15 minutes for 1 hour, then every 30 minutes for 3 hours, then hourly for 20 hours
    C. Every 15 minutes for 2 hours, then every 30 mins for 2 hours, then hourly for 8 hours
    D. Every 15 minutes for 3 hours, then every 30 minutes for 3 hours, then hourly for 3 hours

30. Which medication is *not* indicated for the control of shivering during therapeutic cooling?
    A. Buspirone
    B. Magnesium
    C. Meperidine
    D. Botulinum toxin

8

Medications

ANSWERS

1. **B** Aspirin 81 mg is the only antiplatelet agent with indication for primary prevention (Meschia et al., 2014).

2. **D** The mechanism of action of each antiplatelet agent varies, but they all inactivate different aspects of platelet metabolism, thus inhibiting the normal platelet function. When an injury causes a blood vessel wall to break, platelets are activated, that is, they change shape from round to spiny, stick to the broken vessel wall and to each other, and begin to plug the break. They interact with other blood proteins to form fibrin strands that, in turn, form a net that catches more platelets and blood cells, producing a clot that plugs the break. This function is essential with an injury or surgical incision. The problem is when the innermost lining of blood vessels, the intima, gets roughened by uncontrolled hypertension or uncontrolled diabetes, platelets tend to aggregate along the rough patches of the vessel walls and eventually accumulate, which results in atherosclerosis or thrombus formation (Moake, 2016).

3. **B** Stroke or transient ischemic attack (TIA) patients taking warfarin should not eliminate salads and foods rich in vitamin K, but should be consistent because vitamin K inhibits the action of warfarin. They should

also not be told to limit physical activity as that is an important part of a healthy lifestyle. There is no specific indication for warfarin to be taken with or without food; either is acceptable.

4. **A** Rivaroxaban (Xarelto) can be crushed and administered via a feeding tube, as long as the tube is not in the postpyloric position. Dabigatran should not be crushed; apixaban can be given via a feeding tube but the stomach must be empty as food interferes with the crushed version of this drug. Abciximab is not administered enterally.

5. **A** Alteplase's action is via the promotion of lysis (breaking down) of fibrin clots, also called fibrinolysis.

6. **C** Lisinopril is an angiotensin-converting enzyme inhibitor (ACEI), and combination therapy with alteplase has shown an increased incidence of orolingual angioedema (5%).

7. **C** Lisinopril is an angiotensin-converting enzyme inhibitor (ACEI), and via a complex chemical process, proinflammatory mechanisms occur in the lungs, resulting in a dry cough in up to 20% of patients.

8. **A** In numerous studies, atorvastatin (Lipitor) was compared to placebo, pravastatin, and simvastatin, and was shown to reduce the risk of death or major cardiovascular events more effectively.

9. **D** In numerous studies, IV bolus administration of 23.4% saline has been found to reduce intracranial pressure (ICP) and augment cerebral perfusion pressure (CPP) in patients with resistant increased ICP.

10. **B** Owing to its vasodilation effect, niacin can cause flushing, which can be uncomfortable. Pretreatment with aspirin can be helpful in mitigating this effect.

11. **C** Insulin glargine (Lantus) is a long-acting insulin.

12. **B** Historically, metformin (Glucophage) was held after IV contrast to avoid kidney burden while the contrast was being excreted. Guidelines from 2015 have indicated that this is no longer believed to be a fact, and there should be no need to hold metformin, but it will likely be seen in practice for some time.

13. *A, B, D* Stroke patients are at high risk for depression, so you should never just let this type of comment pass without taking action. Reassure Mr. Smith that his feelings are not unusual, and that he will have help to deal with these feelings. Report this conversation to the provider and monitor Mr. Smith's mood and behavior for further changes.

14. *D* Any of the above; there is no clear advantage of one over the other selective serotonin reuptake inhibitors (SSRIs).

15. *A* It has been shown that antidepressants may enhance neurogenesis and thus functional recovery. There have been suggestions that antidepressants may augment pain therapy, but no clinical trial has shown it to make physical therapy less painful. Antidepressants vary in their effect on appetite, with many actually causing weight gain. For patients with concerns about the stigma of psychiatric medications, it is helpful to point out other benefits of the medications to reassure these patients of physical recovery reasons to justify taking the medications, and that they are not taking them because they are crazy.

16. *A* Fentanyl buccal route is available in oral "lollipop" form.

17. *C* Acetaminophen has a very weak antiplatelet effect, and only at very high doses. Ibuprofen and aspirin have a stronger antiplatelet effect and should not be given periprocedurely.

18. *B* Alteplase (Activase) is the only drug that dissolves blood clots. The others inhibit clot formation, but do not dissolve them.

19. *C* The standard dosing is 0.9 mg/kg over 60 minutes, with 10% of the total dose given as bolus over 1 minute. This patient was 250 lbs, or 113 kgs, but the maximum dose is 90 mg, regardless of weight, so bolus would be 9 mg.

20. *B* Research has shown that antithrombotics given early facilitate better patient outcomes, so you will get an order for a suppository right away. Antithrombotics are not to be given within 24 hours after IV tissue plasminogen activator (tPA) however.

21. *D* Warfarin (Coumadin) is the only anticoagulant to be measured by INR; the use of an INR to determine the effectiveness and safety of the others is meaningless because INR is calibrated for use with vitamin K antagonists.

22. *A* The fact that he started taking gingko for memory help is important because it is an herbal supplement that happens to have several drug interactions, as do many of the herbal supplements. Patients often do not consider them drugs, and may fail to mention that they are using them. Education about this is critical.

23. *A* Dipyridamole/aspirin (Aggrenox) produces headache most frequently in patients with a history of migraine, and can be mitigated with careful dose titration.

24. *C* Lorazepam (Ativan) is considered the first-line agent for treatment of seizure poststroke.

25. *C* Patients with an insulin drip should have their blood glucose monitored every 1 to 2 hours to ensure that the target is maintained and to prevent the extremes of hypoglycemia or hyperglycemia.

26. *D* It was approved by the FDA in 1996 for 3 hours from onset. While many guidelines have recommended that it is safe in select populations up to 4.5 hours from onset, it was not approved by the FDA for that timeframe, so its use in the 3- to 4.5-hour window is considered "off-label."

27. *B* Ten percent of the total dose is given as a bolus over 1 minute. There is no indication for a larger gauge needle. It should not be shaken, but twirled, to mix. If anaphylactic reaction is noted, the drug should be stopped immediately and action taken to treat the anaphylaxis.

28. *B* Oral nimodipine should be administered to all aneurysmal subarachnoid hemorrhage (SAH) patients, a Class I, Level of Evidence A recommendation. It has been shown to improve outcomes, but not necessarily to control vasospasm (Connolly et al., 2012).

29. *A* The schedule for monitoring was defined in 2003 in the first Guidelines for the Early Management of Patients With Ischemic Stroke, and remains today to be every 15 minutes for 2 hours, then every 30 minutes for 6 hours, then hourly for 16 hours.

30. *D* Botulinum toxin is not indicated for controlling of shivering; it is used for treatment of poststroke spasticity.

References

Connolly, E., Rabinstein, A., Carhuapoma, R., Derdeyn, C., Dion, J., Higashida, R. T., . . . Vespa, P. (2012). Guidelines for the management of aneurysmal subarachnoid hemorrhage: A guideline for healthcare professionals from the American Heart Association/American Stroke Association. *Stroke, 43*, 1711–1737.

Meschia, J. F., Bushnell, C., Boden-Albala, B., Braun, L. T., Bravata, D. M., Chaturvedi, S., . . . Wilson, J. A. (2014). Guidelines for the primary prevention of stroke: A statement for healthcare professionals from the American Heart Association/American Stroke Association. *Stroke, 45*, 3754–3832.

Moake, J. L. (2016). How blood clots. *Merck Manual.* Retrieved from https://www.merck manuals.com/home/blood-disorders/blood-clotting-process/how-blood-clots

9

Postacute Care

QUESTIONS

1. Name the leading cause of institutionalization of stroke survivors who had been discharged to go home from the hospital after their stroke.

   A. Noncompliance with medications resulting in complications
   B. Recurrent stroke
   C. New onset seizure disorder
   D. Family members unable to sustain care needs

2. A 70-year-old hemiparetic patient who demonstrates ability to tolerate 3 hours of therapy a day, can eat with assistance, and has two sons who live next door can anticipate which discharge disposition?

   A. Inpatient rehabilitation facility (IRF)
   B. Skilled nursing facility (SNF)
   C. Long-term acute care (LTAC) facility
   D. Home

3. Botulinum toxin injection has proven effective poststroke for which condition?

   A. Urinary incontinence
   B. Focal spasticity

ANSWERS TO THIS SECTION CAN BE FOUND ON PAGE 118

    C. Facial palsy

    D. Balance deficit

4. Your neighbor was discharged to go home after her stroke. When you visit, she tells you that two therapists had come earlier in the day. The first showed her tips on using an adapted spoon for eating cereal/soup, and the second showed her practical tips for using her walker in the house. What types of therapists were they?

    A. Occupational therapist and physical therapist

    B. Recreational therapist and physical therapist

    C. Physical therapist and occupational therapist

    D. Vocational therapist and occupational therapist

5. Which is true of the Barthel Index?

    A. There are 10 items that measure independence and self-care ability

    B. Normal score is 100

    C. It does not adequately quantify disability in high-functioning stroke patients

    D. All of the above

6. Which of the following is also called a subacute rehabilitation facility?

    A. Inpatient rehabilitation facility (IRF)

    B. Skilled nursing facility (SNF)

    C. Long-term acute care hospital (LTACH)

    D. Home health care agency (HHCA)

7. Up to 70% of stroke patients will experience this during the first 6 months after discharge from the hospital or rehabilitation facility:

    A. Shoulder subluxation

    B. Urinary tract infection

    C. Dysphagia

    D. Falling

8. Which is *not* true regarding seizures after an ischemic stroke (Winstein et al., 2016)?

    A. Prophylactic administration of antiepileptic drugs is recommended

    B. Seizures are classified as early (within the first few days) or late

    C. Seizures with lacunar strokes are rare

    D. Seizures are more common in strokes involving the cerebral cortex

9. Which functional measurement tool is the only one used by the Centers for Medicare & Medicaid Services (CMS) related to its prospective payment system?

A. Barthel Index (BI)
B. Functional Independence Measure (FIM®)
C. Modified Rankin Score (mRS)
D. National Institutes of Health Stroke Scale (NIHSS)

10. Your patient, Mr. White, has been in your acute rehabilitation hospital for 1 week now. He continues to eat only the food on the right half of his tray despite his wife's insistence that he should clean his plate. What is your best nursing response to this situation?

A. Establish a behavioral contract with Mr. White that if he finishes his tray completely, he gets an extra dessert
B. Place all his food on the right half of the tray
C. Report this behavior to the provider and suggest a behavioral medicine consult
D. Educate/reeducate the wife and patient about inattention/neglect and reinforce the strategies provided by the occupational therapist

11. After 10 days in the acute rehabilitation hospital, Mrs. Talbot says she just wants to go home to her apartment to her two cats and her canary. The care team has just discussed with her that her progress has not been as much as anticipated. Which of the following would make it more likely that she would be able to go home as she desires?

A. Doubling therapy times for the next week
B. Increasing doses of antidepressant
C. Daughter's ability to move in with her for 6 months
D. Patient's neighbor committing to check on her every day

12. Poststroke spasticity occurs in 25% to 43% of stroke survivors and these patients get aggressive therapy. What is the outcome that these therapies are attempting to prevent?

A. Contractures
B. Hypoperfusion
C. Flaccid limb
D. Wrinkling

13. Your patient had an intracerebral hemorrhage (ICH) 10 days ago. The patient's history of renal failure requiring dialysis and labile hypertension has complicated his hospital stay. The patient is able to participate in therapy services, and has made progress with swallowing, but still requires tube feed support. He is being discharged tomorrow; what is the most likely discharge disposition?

    A. Inpatient rehabilitation facility (IRF)
    B. Assisted living facility
    C. Long-term acute care hospital (LTACH)
    D. Skilled nursing facility (SNF)

14. For Mr. White, a 74-year-old ischemic stroke patient to qualify for home health care, what condition must be present?

    A. He must have supplemental insurance that covers home health care
    B. He must be homebound
    C. He must require at least two therapies and one nursing care need
    D. He must be able to answer the door when the staff arrive

15. In what setting would a physiatrist most likely be employed full time to oversee the functional recovery of a stroke patient?

    A. Inpatient rehabilitation facility (IRF)
    B. Assisted living facility
    C. Home health care agency
    D. Skilled nursing facility (SNF)

16. The role of a rehabilitation nurse in an inpatient rehabilitation facility (IRF) would include

    A. Coordinating care team activities
    B. Reinforcing the care provided by other team members
    C. Advocating for both the client and caregiver
    D. All of the above

17. During his acute rehabilitation stay, Mr. Smith receives cognitive therapy. Which care team member would provide him with this therapy?

    A. Neuropsychologist
    B. Occupational therapist
    C. Speech and language pathologist
    D. All of the above

18. Which of the following is true regarding rehabilitation nurses?

    A. Certification programs for rehabilitation nursing require a bachelor of science in nursing (BSN) and 5 years rehabilitation experience

    B. A 1% increase in the number of certified rehabilitation nurses on a unit is associated with a 6% decrease in length of stay

    C. Rehabilitation nurses provide home visits after discharge from acute rehabilitation

    D. None of the above

19. You suspect that your patient is showing signs of depression. You know this is not uncommon poststroke, and that it is likely the result of which of the following?

    A. Organic, related to the neuronal damage of the stroke

    B. Premorbid, related to having risk factors for depression prior to stroke

    C. Reactive, related to the loss of prestroke independence

    D. All of the above

20. Fecal incontinence and constipation are common after stroke and are attributable to

    A. Polypharmacy resulting in decreased bowel motility

    B. Frequent therapy sessions resulting in irritable bowel

    C. Decreased mobilization and limited access to toilet

    D. Spasticity of the smooth muscles of the bowel

9

Postacute Care

ANSWERS

1. **D** Families care for 74% of stroke survivors after discharge to go home, which takes a terrible toll on the caregivers, with a reported 52% incidence of depression and a 63% higher mortality risk than others their age who are not caregivers (Steiner et al., 2008).

2. **A** The criteria for an inpatient acute rehabilitation stay are the ability to tolerate 3 hours of therapy a day, and a discharge plan that includes support for return to the community (Morrison, 2014, p. 138).

3. **B** Botulinum toxin has been proven effective poststroke for treatment of spasticity. It is a neurotoxin that blocks the chemicals that make muscles tight. The intent of the therapy is to loosen the muscles enough to facilitate physical therapy and recovery of function.

4. **A** Occupational therapists (OTs) help people maximize their independence with an emphasis on useful or functional activities. They help people recover by improving their ability to do day-to-day tasks, also called activities of daily living (ADL). Physical therapists help restore physical functioning and skills such as walking, range of motion, and balance. Recreational therapists help stroke survivors learn strategies to improve the thinking and movement skills needed to join in recreational

activities. Vocational therapists work to help stroke survivors regain skills and develop new skills in order to return to work—either the previous work setting or a new work setting.

5. **D** The Barthel Index is a scale that measures ability to perform 10 self-care and mobility functions. Each function is scored 1 to 10 with a total score of 100, which indicates independence. One criticism is that it is not sensitive enough to quantify disability in high-functioning stroke patients.

6. **B** Skilled nursing facilities (SNFs) have also been referred to as subacute rehabilitation facilities because they provide therapy services for patients who cannot tolerate acute rehabilitation level therapies—so "subacute" (Winstein et al., 2016).

7. **D** Up to 70% of individuals with a stroke experience a fall during the first 6 months after discharge from a hospital or rehabilitation facility. Shoulder subluxation occurs in up to 22% of patients. Urinary tract infection occurs in 10% of patients postdischarge. Dysphagia occurs in up to 30% of stroke patients (Winstein et al., 2016).

8. **A** Patients who have not experienced a seizure poststroke—whether ischemic or hemorrhagic—should not receive prophylactic antiepileptic drugs. Research has not demonstrated that the benefit outweighs the side effects of these drugs.

9. **B** The FIM is an 18-item scale that assesses progress during inpatient rehabilitation along two dimensions: motor (13 items) and cognitive (five items). It evaluates six areas of function: self-care, sphincter control, mobility, locomotion, communication, and social cognition, and is designed to measure one's ability to function with independence (Winstein et al., 2016, p. e114).

10. **D** This patient is exhibiting spatial extinction, or neglect, in which he is unaware of the environment on his left side. The best response is to make sure he and his wife understand why this is happening, and to follow the therapist's recommendations.

11. **C** An important consideration for readiness for discharge from acute rehabilitation is support in the community; for example, a daughter who could move in for a period of time to help.

12. *A* Unresolved spasticity results in contracture of the joint and muscle atrophy, and therapy to relieve the spasticity is aimed at preventing these outcomes.

13. *C* Patients with complex medical needs requiring acute care stays of at least 25 days are discharged to long-term acute care hospitals (LTACHs; Winstein et al., 2016, p. e102).

14. *B* For Medicare patients to qualify for home health care, they must be certified as homebound by a physician (Winstein et al., 2016, p. e102).

15. *A* Physiatrists oversee the functional recovery in acute rehabilitation hospitals.

16. *D* The role of the rehabilitation nurse is in coordination of the care of the interdisciplinary team, reinforcing the care recommendations made by all team members, and advocating for the patient and family throughout the rehabilitation stay (Miller et al., 2010).

17. *D* Each of these members of the care team provides different aspects of cognitive therapy—a strength of a rehabilitation care team that employs all three types of professionals.

18. *B* A study of 54 U.S. rehabilitation facilities found that even a 1% increase in the number of certified rehabilitation nurses on units was associated with a 6% decrease in patient length of stay (Miller et al., 2010, p. 2404).

19. *D* Poststroke depression can occur as a result of the physical damage of the stroke, or as a result of the person's reaction to the effect of the stroke. It is also more likely with people who had a history of risk factors for stroke (Miller et al., 2010).

20. *C* Fecal incontinence and constipation often occur as a result of decreased mobilization and limited access to a toilet. Bowel motility is stimulated by physical activity; many patients will suppress the urge to move their bowels if their only option is a bedpan or bedside commode.

References

Miller, E., Murray, L., Richards, L., Zorowitz, R., Bakas, T., Clark, P., & Billinger, S. (2010). Comprehensive overview of nursing and interdisciplinary rehabilitation care of the stroke patient: A scientific statement from the American Heart Association. *Stroke, 41,* 2402–2048.

Morrison, K. J. (2014). *Fast facts for stroke care nursing: An expert guide in a nutshell.* New York, NY: Springer Publishing.

Steiner, V., Pierce, L., Drahuschak, S., Nofziger, E., Buchman, D., & Szironr, T. (2008). Emotional support, physical help, and health of caregivers of stroke survivors. *Journal of Neuroscience Nursing, 40*(1), 48–54.

Winstein, C. J., Stein, J., Arena, R., Bates, B., Cherney, L. R., Cramer, S. C., . . . Zorowitz, R. D. (2016). Guidelines for adult stroke rehabilitation and recovery: A guideline for healthcare professionals from the American Heart Association/American Stroke Association. *Stroke, 47,* e98–e169.

10

Systems and Quality Care

QUESTIONS

1. The Recommendations for Establishment of Primary Stroke Centers were published in 2001. Who wrote these recommendations?

    A. The Joint Commission (TJC)
    B. American Stroke Association
    C. National Stroke Association
    D. Brain Attack Coalition (BAC)

2. Which of the following cannot provide review and certification of Primary Stroke Centers?

    A. Healthcare Facilities Accreditation Program (HFAP)
    B. Det Norse Veritas (DNV)
    C. National Quality Forum (NQF)
    D. State of Texas

3. Benchmarking refers to the process of

    A. Seeking out best practices and building performance improvement goals to attain them
    B. Comparing your current internal performance data against past performance data, or comparison among nursing units

ANSWERS TO THIS SECTION CAN BE FOUND ON PAGE 127

C. Comparing your facility's aspiration pneumonia rates with those of the stroke centers in your region

D. All of the above

4. Which is *not* true of stroke databases?

   A. Stroke center certification requires use of Microsoft Excel™ for databases

   B. Stroke database content varies and can include a few data points or hundreds of data points

   C. Stroke databases are sometimes homegrown and sometimes external, contracted systems

   D. The advantage of most external databases is the ability to benchmark

5. Which is true of the Plan, Do, Study, Act (PDSA) process?

   A. There must be a specific timeframe determined, with a specific volume of participants or observations for the process to be reliable

   B. An example could be a bedside nurse noting that Mr. X is still having shoulder pain on Day 4. The nurse reviews previous treatments and nursing interventions, agrees with Mr. X of a new approach for today, provides positioning support and back rub, checks back shortly afterward, notes relief of pain and documents that.

   C. It is a single cycle process that supports meeting or exceeding goals

   D. All of the above

6. According to the American Heart Association, which of the following is not a key component of stroke systems of care?

   A. Prehospital care and triage

   B. National Institutes of Health Stroke Scale (NIHSS) certification for nursing staff

   C. Stroke center certification

   D. Rehabilitation strategies

7. Hospitals with the capability to perform mechanical endovascular reperfusion (MER) would have which stroke center certification?

   A. Primary Stroke Center (PSC)

   B. Comprehensive Stroke Center (CSC)

   C. Acute Stroke Ready Hospital (ASRH)

   D. Either PSC or CSC

8. A key distinction between Comprehensive Stroke Center (CSC) and Primary Stroke Center (PSC) is which of the following?

   A. 24/7 MRI/magnetic resonance angiography (MRA)
   B. Neurocritical care unit led by neurocritical care specialist
   C. The ability to mix and administer IV tissue plasminogen activator (tPA) in less than 60 minutes
   D. The ability to care for hemorrhagic stroke patients

9. Clinical practice guidelines can most accurately be described as

   A. Statements that include recommendations to optimize care, that are informed by a systematic review of evidence
   B. Recommendations that have been approved by the American Heart Association/American Stroke Association
   C. Order sets based on the preferences of the stroke neurologist or vascular neurosurgeon
   D. Recommendations provided by The Joint Commission after a certification visit

10. Which of the following are the benefits of having a stroke unit where the majority of stroke patients are cared for? (Choose all that apply.)

   A. Reduced in-hospital mortality
   B. Reduced bladder incontinence
   C. Reduced length of stay
   D. Increased discharges to home

11. As the stroke program coordinator, you have noticed a trend of increased door-to-needle times over the past quarter. The consistent factor that stands out is the involvement of a new emergency department (ED) provider, Dr. X, who has been vocal in her "disapproval" of the use of tissue plasminogen activator (tPA). The ED nurses have described being berated and bullied if they attempt to activate a stroke alert while Dr. X is on duty. What is your best action?

   A. Discuss this situation with all the ED nurses and reassure them that Dr. X is incorrect and outdated in her opinion
   B. Ask the ED medical director to limit Dr. X's involvement in stroke patient cases

    C. Present data to your program medical director and suggest they review with Dr. X

    D. At next stroke alert, ask Dr. X why she does not like tPA

12. The reduction in stroke mortality in the United States has been attributed to many factors. Which one of them has been credited with the broadest impact?

    A. Reduced salt intake

    B. Treatment of hypertension

    C. Reduced soda consumption

    D. Treatment of diabetes

13. The definition of transient ischemic attack (TIA) has evolved from its original definition of any focal cerebral ischemic event with symptoms lasting less than 24 hours. What is the reason for the change in definition to a tissue-based criterion rather than a time-based criterion?

    A. Laboratory testing on animal models

    B. Retrospective review of records from large academic medical centers

    C. Enhanced imaging capabilities enabling more accurate identification of infarct even with symptom resolution in under 24 hours

    D. None of the above

14. There are many standards and metrics for stroke center certification. The key feature of a successful stroke center is

    A. Collection, analysis, and use of data for performance improvement

    B. Administrative support

    C. Appropriate and up-to-date order sets, protocols, and policies

    D. Annual staff education and competency documentation

15. One of your stroke patients was found unconscious on the floor of the bathroom, with a fresh scalp laceration. An in-depth internal review of all factors related to this event is being conducted. Which type of performance improvement process is being used?

    A. Plan, Do, Study, Act (PDSA)

    B. Six Sigma

    C. Define, Measure, Analyze, Improve, Control (DMAIC)

    D. Root cause analysis

Systems and Quality Care

ANSWERS

1. **D** The BAC was established in 1991 by a group of neurosurgeons who saw the opportunity to improve stroke care through standardization and evidence-based guidelines. They were inspired by the improved patient outcomes seen with trauma guidelines. It includes members from 17 professional organizations including the American Association of Neuroscience Nurses. In 2003, TJC started its Primary Stroke Center certification process as part of its Disease-Specific Care certification program. Many people have credited TJC with creating the standards for Primary Stroke Centers, but in fact it was the BAC (Morrison, 2014).

2. **C** The NQF is a not-for-profit, nonpartisan, membership-based organization that works to facilitate improvements in health care, but it does not have certifying authority. HFAP and DNV are certifying organizations in competition with TJC. There are also many states that have their own stroke center certification program, and Texas is one of them.

3. **D** Benchmarking is a term used to describe all the actions in A, B, and C. It has proven to be a valuable tool in driving performance improvement efforts in hospitals (Ettorchi-Tardy, Levif, & Michel, 2012).

4. *A* The term "stroke database" is used to describe a wide variety of stroke data repositories. Stroke certification only requires that some method of data collection, analysis, and reporting is demonstrated.

5. *B* The PDSA is also referred to as the Plan-Do-Check-Act (PDCA). It is a multicycle process for instituting a new treatment, process, and so on, and then evaluating, adjusting, and repeating the process. It can be done on a large scale with a formal research idea, or in everyday nursing care as described in the question.

6. *B* The American Heart Association's stroke systems of care involve key elements of care across the continuum, based on the standards related to stroke center certification, prehospital collaboration, and rehabilitation care. It does not dictate specifics such as National Institutes of Health Stroke Scale (NIHSS) certification for nursing staff (Higashida et al., 2013).

7. *D* While CSC certification has MER capability as a standard, there are many PSCs with MER capability as well, who may not meet all the CSC standards, but are capable of MER. ASRHs are focused on the emergency department (ED)—identification, stabilization, treatment with IV tissue plasminogen activator (tPA), and transfer to a PSC or CSC.

8. *B* Neurocritical care units led by neurocritical care specialists is an essential standard for CSCs; PSCs can manage hemorrhagic stroke patients, should have MRI 24/7, as well as mix and administer IV tPA in under 60 minutes.

9. *A* Clinical practice guidelines are provided by a variety of expert organizations, not just the American Heart Association/American Stroke Association. They are based on research evidence and guide care of specific populations. They are *not* simply a compilation of provider preference for care.

10. *A, C, D* Evidence published in 1997 demonstrated a 28% reduction in mortality, an 8% reduction in length of stay, and a 7% increase in discharge to home for patients cared for in a dedicated stroke unit (Langhorne et al., 1997).

11. *C* Historically the ED providers' professional organizations, such as the American Academy of Emergency Medicine (AAEM) and the American

College of Emergency Physicians (ACEP), have been opposed to IV tPA on the premise that the studies done to get it approved by the U.S. Food and Drug Administration (FDA) were flawed. So it has been a common occurrence for ED providers to be less than enthusiastic about this drug. The best thing to do is to use peer influence, and support your medical director's speaking with this provider.

12. *B* Progressive treatment and more effective antihypertensive medications has led to a significant impact on the ability to control hypertension, leading to better outcomes (Mozaffarian, 2015).

13. *C* Improved CT and MRI imaging has made it possible to see even miniscule infarcts. Now events lasting less than 24 hours that used to be labeled TIA are often found to be tiny strokes.

14. *A* While all of these choices are part of stroke center certification, the key element is the use of data to drive process improvement, with improved outcomes as well.

15. *D* Root cause analysis is the process of taking an event, usually an adverse outcome, and analyzing every aspect that led up to it to find the cause. The purpose is to then make sure that it does not happen again. DMAIC refers to a data-driven improvement cycle used for improving, optimizing, and stabilizing processes. The DMAIC improvement cycle is the core tool used to drive Six Sigma projects. Six Sigma is a disciplined, data-driven approach and methodology for eliminating defects in any process.

References

Ettorchi-Tardy, A., Levif, M., & Michel, P. (2012). Benchmarking: A method for continuous quality improvement in healthcare. *Healthcare Policy, 7*(4), e101–e119. Retrieved from https://www.ncbi.nlm.nih.gov/pmc/articles/PMC3359088

Higashida, R., Alberts, M. J., Alexander, D. N., Crocco, T. J., Demaerschalk, B. M., Derdeyn, C. P., . . . Wood, J. P. (2013). Interactions within stroke systems of care: A policy statement from the American Heart Association/American Stroke Association. *Stroke, 44*, 2961–2984.

Langhorne, P., Asplund, K., Berman, P., Blomstrand, C., Dennis, M., Douglas, J., . . . Wilhelmsen, L. (1997). Collaborative systematic review of the randomised trials of organised inpatient (stroke unit) care after stroke. *British Medical Journal, 314*, 1151–1158.

Morrison, K. J. (2014). *Fast facts for stroke care nursing: An expert guide in a nutshell.* New York, NY: Springer Publishing.

Mozaffarian, D., Benjamin, E. J., Go, A. S., Arnett, D. K., Blaha, M. J., Cushman M., . . . Turner, M. B. (2015). Heart disease and stroke statistics—2016 update: A report from the American Heart Association. *Circulation, 133,* e38–e360. doi:10.1161/CIR.0000000000000350

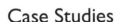

Case Studies

Alicia M. Richardson

QUESTIONS

Prehospital and Emergency Department

Questions 1 and 2 are based on the following case:
Bill Black, a 65-year-old patient, had his symptom onset witnessed by his daughter to be at 9:00 a.m.; it is now 12:30 p.m. His medical history includes heart failure and diabetes. Emergency medical services (EMS) reported a blood glucose of 188.

1. You receive an order for IV tissue plasminogen activator (tPA) to be administered to Mr. Black. Which of the following is correct?

   A. You proceed with administration knowing it is safe to give as ordered
   B. You withhold the drug and notify the provider of the exclusion criteria for the extended time window
   C. You wait for lab glucose results to confirm the EMS report
   D. You review the patient's past medical record, note that HgA1c last year was less than 6, and therefore administer tPA

ANSWERS TO THIS SECTION CAN BE FOUND ON PAGE 142

2. At 1:02 p.m. the decision is made to transfer Mr. Black to a Comprehensive Stroke Center for possible thrombectomy. How much time remains in the window for initiation of endovascular intervention for anterior territory stroke?

   A. Approximately 2 hours
   B. Approximately 4 hours
   C. Approximately 8 hours
   D. Approximately 20 hours

Questions 3 to 6 are based on the following case:
The Southeast emergency medical services (EMS) crew brings Mr. Smith, age 82 years, to the emergency department (ED) on a stretcher. He has become lethargic, is snoring loudly, and slumped to the right. They report his last blood pressure (BP) to be 177/86, heart rate (HR) 90, respiratory rate (RR) 22. They also report right upper extremity weakness and difficulty speaking. His Glasgow Coma Scale (GCS) is 3. Home medications include dabigatran, atorvastatin, and levothyroxine.

3. Which is your first action?

   A. Obtain an EKG
   B. Prepare to intubate
   C. Straighten Mr. Smith's posture
   D. Draw lab work

4. Mr. Smith's CT showed intracerebral hemorrhage (ICH), and the provider ordered coagulation correction. What do you expect to administer?

   A. 20 mL prothrombin complex concentrate (PCC) IV
   B. 2 units fresh frozen plasma (FFP) IV
   C. 10 mg vitamin K IV
   D. 5 g idarucizumab (Praxbind) IV

5. Mr. Smith is getting restless, trying to pull out his IV, and swinging his arms at you. You are concerned when the provider orders lorazepam because

   A. You doubt you can get close enough to administer it without getting hit
   B. You are concerned about drug dependency
   C. You noted a long list of medication allergies on his chart, and wonder if this was on it
   D. You know it will make further neurologic assessments more difficult

6. You are present when the provider calculates Mr. Smith's ICH score. His score is 3. Which of the following is not true of the ICH score?

   A. It includes Glasgow Coma Scale score
   B. It includes age
   C. The score is predictive of 30-day mortality risk
   D. It is based on history of diabetes

In the Intensive Care Unit

Questions 7 to 11 are based on the following case:
Mr. Dobbs is a 66-year-old male who had a left middle cerebral artery (MCA) stroke 2 days ago for which he received IV tissue plasminogen activator (tPA) and mechanical thrombectomy. He has a history of hypertension, and remote cigarette smoking, having quit 5 years ago.

7. You are told that Mr. Dobbs had a thrombolysis in cerebral infarction (TICI) score of 2a with his thrombectomy. What does this indicate about the success of the procedure?

   A. It was only partially successful, with less than two thirds of vascular territory perfused
   B. It was only partially successful, but more successful than a 2b result
   C. It was not successful at all
   D. It was a complete success with over 85% reperfusion

8. The interventionalist indicates that Mr. Dobb's carotid artery was very stenotic and made it difficult to perform the mechanical thrombectomy. What options does the interventionalist have in this type of case?

   A. Angioplasty and stenting
   B. Using the contralateral anterior cerebral artery
   C. Obtain a stat lipid panel
   D. Use the vertebral arteries

9. While out of bed in a chair, Mr. Dobbs demonstrates increased difficulty with having a conversation with his wife, and increased difficulty with feeding himself. What do you suspect is occurring?

   A. Mr. Dobbs is overtired from the exertion of getting out of bed after a long physical therapy/occupational therapy session
   B. Mr. Dobbs is hypoxic as the brain does not store oxygen, but demands more with exertion

    C. Mr. Dobbs is experiencing postural hypotension causing exacerbation of stroke symptoms

    D. Mr. Dobbs is showing signs of depression and cognitive decline

10. Your response to this observation is to get Mr. Dobbs back into bed immediately because you know that

    A. Stroke patients require more rest than most people

    B. Stroke patients can have their cerebral autoregulation impaired making them much more susceptible to deterioration with extreme highs and lows of blood pressure (BP)

    C. When Mr. Dobbs gets this depressed, he does not cooperate or eat well

    D. The oxygen tubing does not reach from the wall source to the chair

11. You check Mr. Dobbs's blood pressure (BP), pulse, and temperature: BP = 120/80, pulse = 84, temperature = 38°C. You take which of the following actions?

    A. Notify the provider and prepare the patient for a stat MRI and a fluid bolus

    B. Ask Mr. Dobbs if he is feeling better, position them in 30° semi-Fowler's position, and administer PRN acetaminophen

    C. Explain to Mr. Dobbs why you needed to get him back into bed quickly, and apply low-dose oxygen

    D. Ensure that the head of the bed is flat, administer PRN acetaminophen, and notify the provider

Questions 12 to 17 are based on the following case:
You are caring for Mr. Booth, a 72-year-old subarachnoid hemorrhage (SAH) patient with a saccular anterior cerebral artery aneurysm found on CT angiogram. On admission his Hunt and Hess score was 2. Today is Day 2 of his stay and his National Institutes of Health Stroke Scale (NIHSS) score is 1—drowsy. His medical history includes type 2 diabetes and hypertension for which he took metformin, aspirin, and lisinopril prior to admission. He is scheduled for an endovascular coiling procedure tomorrow (Day 3). His wife and two brothers are visiting now.

12. As you enter the room, you find Mrs. Booth gently tucking a second blanket up under Mr. Booth's chin and commenting that the draft she feels might give him a chill. What is your best response?

    A. Say nothing and when she leaves, remove the blanket to avoid hyperthermia
    B. Apologize for any discomfort they may have experienced and facilitate a therapeutic environment by increasing the temperature
    C. Explain that hyperthermia is something to be avoided in his case and ask her to help by not putting extra blankets on his bed
    D. Say nothing, but administer acetaminophen 650 mg with his next medication

13. Mrs. Booth expresses concern over the scheduled procedure for tomorrow, asking why it cannot wait until he is more wide awake. What should you include in your response?

    A. A detailed list of all possible treatment options and their success/complication rates
    B. An explanation that research evidence supports treatment as early as possible in order to reduce the risk of rebleed
    C. A suggestion that she ask her primary care provider (PCP) to prescribe something to relax her as she seems overanxious
    D. A reminder that she should have been present at morning rounds in order to ask the doctor that question

14. Mrs. Booth overhears you administering Mr. Booth's morning medications. She questions the drug nimodipine and asks for an explanation of why that was started. You explain by stating that

    A. This medication was added to help control his blood pressure
    B. This is to prevent vasospasms following a subarachnoid hemorrhage
    C. It is to help shrink the size of the aneurysm
    D. It will be discontinued 24 hours after his procedure

15. What does a Hunt and Hess score of 2 indicate about Mr. Booth's situation?

    A. That he was asymptomatic on presentation
    B. That he has intraventricular extension of hemorrhage

    C. That he has two distinct areas of subarachnoid hemorrhage

    D. That he presented with moderate to severe headache, but no focal neurologic deficits

16. Mrs. Booth asks what to expect when her husband returns from his procedure tomorrow. What do you tell her?

    A. He will probably be more sleepy and will be having his vital signs and groin checked frequently for several hours

    B. There should be no difference in his condition or routine noted

    C. He will go to the stroke unit immediately postprocedure; no need for the intensive care unit (ICU) once an aneurysm is secured

    D. He will likely be intubated with multiple IV fluids infusing for support of cerebral perfusion pressure

17. When you check Mr. Booth's vital signs, you note a rise in systolic blood pressure (SBP) from 138 to 148, with no change in pulse rate or temperature. Your next action should be which of the following?

    A. Assess for neurologic change and recheck BP

    B. Explain the importance of keeping the environment quiet and calm and ask visitors to leave

    C. Notify the provider and prepare for stat CT scan

    D. Both A and B

Questions 18 to 22 are based on the following case:

Ms. Clark is a 23-year-old intracerebral hemorrhage (ICH) patient who was admitted yesterday after being found on the floor at work. She was awake but dazed on admission, with an ICH score of 1, and an National Institutes of Health Stroke Scale (NIHSS) score of 0, Glasgow Coma Scale (GCS) score of 15. Her medical history includes only smoking 1 to 2 packs/day for the past 8 years. Imaging has revealed a moderate subcortical arteriovenous malformation (AVM) in the right temporal lobe. She has a family history of her maternal grandmother dying from a brain hemorrhage—cause unknown. The next five questions pertain to this case.

18. What components are involved in the intracerebral hemorrhage (ICH) score?

    A. Glasgow Coma Scale

    B. ICH volume

C. Age

D. All of the above

19. What does the intracerebral hemorrhage (ICH) score of 1 tell you about Ms. Clark's prognosis?

A. She has a high likelihood of dying from her stroke within 30 days

B. She may survive but with a high likelihood of disability

C. She has a high likelihood of surviving her stroke

D. She is lucky to have arrived at the hospital alive

20. Which complication will you most likely see with this patient?

A. Aspiration pneumonia

B. Seizures

C. Urinary tract infection

D. Skin breakdown

21. By the end of Day 2 Ms. Clark has become less responsive and has required intubation. There is also concern for rising intracranial pressure (ICP). Her systemic blood pressure (BP) has been 130 to 140/82 to 88, temperature 37.8°C. Which procedure do you anticipate being done next?

A. Insertion of nasogastric tube for enteral feeding

B. Initiation of therapeutic hypothermia

C. Placement of ventricular catheter for cerebrospinal fluid (CSF) drainage

D. Stat craniotomy for clot evacuation

22. In addition to monitoring her blood pressure and intracranial pressure (ICP) what other clinical parameters are critical for the ICU nurse to monitor and control?

A. Blood glucose and temperature

B. Creatinine and Hgb A1c

C. INR and partial thromboplastin time (PTT)

D. Pupil size and bowel sounds

Postacute Care

Questions 23 to 27 are based on the following case:

Your rehabilitation patient, Mr. Phillips, is a 78-year-old widower who has upper extremity and gait training needs, two of the most common

interventions provided during inpatient rehabilitation. He has been at rehabilitation for 8 days and has been making progress with therapy. His tenta-
tive discharge plan is home with 24-hour family assistance.

23. His daughter arrived from out of state and asks you why his unaffected
arm is in a sling for several hours a day. What is your best response?

   A. It is a technique used to prevent him from pulling out his nasogastric
   (NG) tube
   B. By reducing muscle strength of the unaffected side, the affected side
   is forced to get stronger
   C. It is a technique to increase his desire to be independent
   D. Constraint-induced movement therapy, a highly studied technique,
   involves limitation of the unaffected arm for controlled lengths of
   time each day in order to encourage use of the affected arm

24. His daughter attends therapy sessions with Mr. Phillips and has another
question for you the next day. What is your best response to her question
about why he has shoulder pain?

   A. Shoulder pain can occur with upper extremity paresis as a result of
   the weight of the limb and reduced muscle, ligament, and tendon
   function around the shoulder.
   B. He may have fallen and injured his arm, but he did not report anything and no one witnessed a fall
   C. Rehabilitation hospital beds are not very comfortable for tall
   patients and as Mr. Phillips is over 6 feet tall, that may result in some
   discomfort
   D. Pain is a common result of stroke, and the location of the pain is
   dependent on the area of the brain affected

25. Mr. Phillips's daughter then asks you what will be done about this shoulder pain. What is your best response?

   A. Staff are trained to avoid pulling on the affected arm when assisting
   him out of bed
   B. Staff are trained to ensure proper support/positioning of the affected
   arm while in a chair, bed, or ambulating
   C. Pain medication is provided
   D. All of the above

26. Mr. Phillips asks why the therapist makes him walk on the treadmill every day. What is your best response?

A. Burning calories will help prevent weight gain, a common challenge for stroke survivors

B. Treadmill training has been shown to improve endurance, gait, and to promote cortical reorganization

C. Treadmill training will soon be replaced by robot-assisted therapy, but it is not available yet

D. Treadmill training is really focused on making Mr. Phillips use his affected upper extremity for support without realizing it

27. Mr. Phillips is nearing discharge and his daughter is concerned about his transition to home. She lives out of state and heard he needs 24-hour supervision that she cannot provide. What should you tell her?

A. A skilled nursing facility is a better discharge disposition

B. She could take advantage of the Family and Medical Leave Act (FMLA) and provide the care he needs at home

C. You will request a family meeting with care coordination and social work

D. 24-hour supervision is only a suggestion and he can still go home

Preventive Care

Questions 28 to 32 are based on the following case:
You are working with the acute care team in preparation of the discharge plan for Mr. Moore, a 60-year-old divorced man who has had a third stroke, etiology of small vessel disease. It is Day 3 and his National Institutes of Health Stroke Scale (NIHSS) score is 3—he has aphasia (1) and motor weakness (1) and sensory loss (1) of his right upper extremity. His medical history includes diabetes, hypertension, depression, and remote history of cigarette smoking, having quit 2 years ago. His Hgb A1c is 8, and his blood pressure (BP) has been 140 to 158/78 to 88.

28. In your routine assessment, you note that Mr. Moore seems gloomy and quiet compared to yesterday, and you report this to the care team on rounds. What action can you expect?

A. Stat psychiatric consult

B. Review of home medications for antidepressant and discuss with Mr. Moore

C. If on antidepressants already, change of medication

D. Suicide precautions

29. Mr. Moore offers you some chocolate from his secret stash that he says he keeps for when he needs something sweet. He asks you not to tell his doctor. What do you do?

   A. Remind Mr. Moore that with his history of diabetes he should not have chocolate and the candy should be sent home with his family when they visit

   B. To keep Mr. Moore from eating them, remove them when he is asleep and share them with the nurses. If he asks about them, tell him it was for his own good

   C. Explain that his Hgb A1c was high on admission, which indicates poor control of his diabetes over the past few months, and if he does not get that under control he is likely to keep having strokes. Offer to keep the candy for him until his family arrives so that he is not tempted

   D. Scold him for cheating and make him watch while you flush them down the toilet

30. When Mr. Moore complains about having to change his blood pressure (BP) medication because of just having had a 6-month supply delivered to his house last week. You respond in what way?

   A. Remind him that he should feel lucky to only have had a mild stroke, and without divulging names, tell him about the patient in the next room who had a major stroke

   B. Empathize with him, and show him his BP trend explaining that this medical regimen is keeping his BP exactly where it needs to be which should reduce his risk of another stroke

   C. Empathize with him and talk with him about the sorry state of affairs our health care system is in

   D. Explain that in a few months, he should be able to work his way back to using these medications

31. During your education about lifestyle choices that will improve chances of better health, Mr. Moore tells you that he takes a 60-minute brisk walk

every Monday, Wednesday, Friday, and Saturday. He asks if he should increase this level of activity. What would be your answer?

A. Ask him if he was an athlete in high school, and recommend he review what his activity level was at his peak

B. Recommend adding another aerobic activity on Tuesday, Thursday, and Sunday to avoid being sedentary those days

C. He should consider increasing from brisk walk to running since he had a stroke at this level of activity

D. This level of activity exceeds the recommendations of the American Heart Association/American Stroke Association, so he does not need to increase

32. The therapists have recommended that Mr. Moore should have outpatient speech and occupational therapy after discharge. You overhear Mr. Moore tell his son that he does not intend to keep those appointments because of the high copays. What do you do?

A. Inform the care team and document that he is noncompliant with his plan of care

B. Ask the care manager and therapists to try to get him charity care

C. Ask the therapists to discuss the anticipated number of therapy sessions needed and the options for teaching him exercises to do on his own

D. Tell him that he probably does not need any more structured therapy as he has shown some improvement already

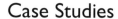

Case Studies

Alicia M. Richardson

ANSWERS

Prehospital and Emergency Department

1. **A** The patient is in the extended window (up to 4.5 hours) for administration of tPA according to the last known well time. Exclusion criteria in the extended window include patients older than 80 years, history of stroke and diabetes, and international normalized ratio (INR) higher than 1.7 regardless of taking Coumadin. This patient meets the criteria for extended window and therefore it is safe to administer tPA (Del Zoppo, Saver, Jauch, & Adams, 2009).

2. **A** Based on the American Heart Association/American Stroke Association 2015 endovascular treatment guidelines, initiation of endovascular therapy should occur within 6 hours from onset for best outcome. At the time of transfer decision, this patient is already 4 hours into his window, therefore there is only approximately 2 hours left (Powers et al., 2015).

3. **B** With a GCS of 3, lethargy, and snoring, it is important to recognize that the first action should be to stabilize an airway and intubate this patient.

4. **D** The patient is taking dabigatran (Pradaxa) and the reversal agent is idarucizumab (Praxbind).

5. **D** Benzodiazepines should be avoided in patients with neurologic impairment as it will make further neurologic assessment more difficult.

6. **D** The ICH score is comprised of age, GCS, location, ICH volume, and the presence of intraventricular blood. The score is predictive of 30-day mortality risk (Morrison, 2014).

In the Intensive Care Unit

7. **A** The TICI score is used to measure the postreperfusion obtained after a mechanical thrombectomy. A TICI of 0: no perfusion; TICI 1: antegrade reperfusion past the initial occlusion, but limited distal branch filling with little or slow distal reperfusion; TICI 2: antegrade reperfusion of less than half of the occluded target artery previously ischemic territory (e.g., in one major division of the MCA and its territory); TICI 2B: antegrade reperfusion of more than half of the previously occluded target artery ischemic territory (e.g., in two major divisions of the MCA and their territories); TICI 3: complete antegrade reperfusion of the previously occluded target artery ischemic territory, with absence of visualized occlusion in all distal branches (Fugate, Klunder, & Kallmes, 2013).

8. **A** Angioplasty and stenting are often used in cases where carotid stenosis is present.

9. **C** Stroke symptoms can return when out of bed or during activity, as some patients are perfusion dependent, especially if they have carotid disease. This patient is likely having postural hypotension, which is exacerbating stroke symptoms (Morrison, 2014, p. 115).

10. **B** Stroke patients have cerebral autoregulation impairment and therefore cannot tolerate extreme fluctuations in their blood pressure, otherwise stroke symptoms may return (Morrison, 2014, p. 115).

11. **D** In order to correct perfusion-dependent hypotension, this patient should be returned to bed, with the head of the bed flat to increase the perfusion to the brain. It is also important to maintain normothermia and administer acetaminophen (Tylenol) as needed (Morrison, 2014, pp. 110–115).

12. **C** Normothermia should be maintained in patients with stroke; hyperthermia should be avoided as it has been associated with a two fold increase in short-term mortality. The patient should have excess blankets removed, and be given acetaminophen (Tylenol) as needed to maintain normothermia (Morrison, 2014, p. 111).

13. **B** In patients with aneurysmal SAH, it is important to secure the aneurysm as soon as possible in order to reduce the risk of rebleeding (Morrison, 2014, p. 90).

14. **B** Nimodipine is the first-line drug for the prevention of vasospasm in SAH patients. It should be administered within the first 24 hours and until the patient is outside the vasospasm window.

15. **D** The Hunt and Hess is a severity scale used in SAH patients: a score of 1: mild headache, alert and oriented, minimal nuchal rigidity; score of 2: full nuchal rigidity, moderate to severe headache, alert and oriented, no neurologic deficit; score of 3: lethargy or confusion, mild focal neurologic deficits; score 4: stuporous, more severe focal deficits; score 5: comatose, showing signs of severe neurologic impairment (e.g., posturing).

16. **A** Postaneurysm repair patients will require frequent vital signs, neurologic checks, and groin site checks. They may be drowsy following the procedure if they received anesthesia (Morrison, 2014, p. 126).

17. **D** The postintervention environment should be kept calm and quiet with frequent monitoring of BP and neurologic checks (Morrison, 2014, p. 126).

18. **D** The ICH score is comprised of age, GCS, location, ICH volume and the presence of intraventricular blood. The score is predictive of 30-day mortality risk (Morrison, 2014).

19. **C** The score is predictive of 30-day mortality risk and the lower the score the less risk associated and higher likelihood of survival (Morrison, 2014).

20. **B** Seizure is a common complication to assess for in ICH population.

21. **C** Patients with worsening neurologic examinations and increasing ICP may require a ventricular catheter for CSF drainage.

22. *A* Stroke outcomes have been associated with management of temperature, blood glucose, and BP, and therefore it is important to monitor and control these clinical parameters (Morrison, 2014, p. 101).

Postacute Care

23. *B* Constraint-induced movement therapy (CIMT) is where the unaffected arm is placed in a restrictive mitt to encourage use of the weak upper limb; classic therapy involves 6 hours, 5 days per week for a 2-week period (Morrison, 2014, p. 149).

24. *A* Shoulder subluxation can occur in the affected arm of a stroke patient because of the weight of the arm, reduced muscle, and limited ligament and tendon function (Morrison, 2014, p. 116).

25. *D* Treatments for pain associated with shoulder subluxation should include staff training to avoid pulling on the affected arm when assisting the patient out of bed; staff training to ensure proper support and positioning of the affected arm while in a chair, bed, or ambulating: and pain medication as needed (Morrison, 2014, p. 116).

26. *C* Treadmill training improves endurance, gait, and promotes cortical reorganization (Miller et al., 2010).

27. *B* The plan of care needs to be established with care coordination, social work, and the patient/family to enhance successful transition of care and a safe discharge disposition (Morrison, 2014, p. 138).

Preventive Care

28. *B* Review of home medications and discussion with the patient are the best first steps; it is too soon for a psychiatric consult or to make medication changes or suicide precautions.

29. *C* High Hgb A1c indicates a sustained high blood sugar for at least a few months. Persistent hyperglycemia results in vascular damage and needs to be addressed to bring down the risk of many vascular diseases that can result.

30. *B* Empathy is valuable in the setting of medication changes and the practical side of cost. But education about the need for consistent control

of hypertension is an important measure to reduce that risk of vascular disease that can result.

31. *D* Guidelines have changed over the years, and the current recommendations are for moderate to vigorous activity 40 min/day, 3 to 4 times/week. Numerous studies have shown that physically active men and women generally have a 25% to 30% lower risk of stroke or mortality than the least active (Meschia et al., 2014).

32. *C* Copays for therapy appointments are often costly and can be a hard-stop barrier for many patients. Of these choices, the best option would be to at least ensure that he gets information about the anticipated number of sessions and proper instructions from the therapist.

References

Del Zoppo, G. J., Saver, J. L., Jauch, E. C., & Adams, H. P. (2009). Expansion of the time window for treatment of acute ischemic stroke with intravenous tissue plasminogen activator: A science advisory from the American Heart Association/American Stroke Association. *Stroke, 40,* 2945–2948.

Fugate, J. E., Klunder, A. M., & Kallmes, D. F. (2013). What is meant by "TICI"? *American Journal of Neuroradiology, 34*(9), 1792–1797. doi:10.3174/ajnr.A3496

Meschia, J. F., Bushnell, C., Boden-Albala, B., Braun, L. T., Bravata, D. M., Chaturvedi, S., . . . Wilson, J. A. (2014). Guidelines for the primary prevention of stroke: A statement for healthcare professionals from the American Heart Association/American Stroke Association. *Stroke, 45,* 3754–3832.

Miller, E., Murray, L., Richards, L., Zorowitz, R., Bakas, T., Clark, P., & Billinger, S. A. (2010). Comprehensive overview of nursing and interdisciplinary rehabilitation care of the stroke patient: A scientific statement from the American Heart Association. *Stroke, 41,* 2402–2048.

Morrison, K. J. (2014). *Fast facts for stroke care nursing: An expert guide in a nutshell.* New York, NY: Springer Publishing.

Powers, W. J., Derdeyn, C. P., Biller, J., Coffey, C. S., Hoh, B. L., Jauch, E. C., . . . Yavagal, D. R. (2015). 2015 American Heart Association/American Stroke Association focused update of the 2013 guidelines for the early management of patients with acute ischemic stroke regarding endovascular treatment: A guideline for healthcare professionals from the American Heart Association/American Stroke Association. *Stroke, 46,* 3020–3035.

Appendix A: Medications List

Generic Name	Trade Name
Analgesics	
Fentanyl	Duragesic
Oxycodone	Oxycontin, Roxicodone
Morphine	MS Contin, Duramorph
Hydrocodone/Acetaminophen	Vicodin, Lortab
Hydromorphone	Dilaudid
Analgesics/Antipyretics	
Acetaminophen	Tylenol
Ibuprofen	Advil, Motrin
Acetyl Salicylic Acid	Aspirin, Ascriptin, Durlaza, Ecotrin, Ecpirin, Fasprin, Halfprin, Miniprin
Anticonvulsants	
Lorazepam	Ativan
Diazepam	Valium
Phenytoin	Dilantin
Fosphenytoin	Cerebyx
Valproic Acid	Depokene, Stavzor, Depacon, Valproate sodium
Levetiracetam	Keppra
Lacosamide	Vimpat
Pentobarbital	Nembutal

(*continued*)

(continued)

Generic Name	Trade Name
Antidepressants	
Fluoxetine	Prozac
Paroxetine	Paxil
Sertraline	Zoloft
Citalopram	Celexa
Escitalopram	Lexapro
Nortriptyline	Pamelor
Amitriptyline	Elavil
Trazodone	Desyrel
Antihypertensives	
Angiotensin-II Blockers (generic name ends in -artan)	
Valsartan	Diovan
Losartan	Cozaar
Angiotensin Converting Enzyme (ACE) Inhibitors (generic name ends in -pril)	
Enalapril	Vasotec
Lisinopril	Prinivil, Zestril
Benazepril	Lotensin
Captopril	Capoten
Fosinopril	Monopril
Quinapril	Accupril
Ramipril	Altace
Perindopril	Aceon
Beta Blockers (generic name ends in -lol)	
Labetalol	Trandate
Metoprolol	Lopressor
Esmolol	Brevibloc
Acebutolol	Sectral
Atenolol	Tenormin
Nadolol	Corgard
Calcium Channel Blockers (generic name ends in -pine)	
Nicardipine	Cardene

(continued)

(*continued*)

Generic Name	Trade Name
Antihypertensives (*continued*)	
Clevidipine	Cleviprex
Nifedipine	Adalat, Procardia
Nimodipine	Nimotop
Felodipine	Plendil
Diuretics	
Hydrochlorothiazide	Hydrodiuril
Chlorthalidone	Hygroton
Indapamide	Lozol
Furosemide	Lasix
Bumetanide	Bumex
Torsemide	Demadex
Spironolactone	Aldactone
Other Calcium Channel Blockers	
Diltiazem	Cardizem, Tiazac
Verapamil	Calan, Verelan
Vasodilators	
Hydralazine	Apresoline
Nitroglycerin	Nitrostat, NitroQuick, Nitro-Dur, Nitro-Bid
Nitroprusside	Nitropress, Nipride
Fenoldopam	Corlopam
Antispasmodics	
Baclofen	Lioresal
Tizanidine	Zanaflex
Dantrolene	Dantrium
Botulinum Toxin A	Botox
Antithrombotics	
Anticoagulants	
Warfarin	Coumadin
Dabigatran	Pradaxa
Rivaroxaban	Xarelto

(*continued*)

(*continued*)

Generic Name	Trade Name
Antithrombotics (*continued*)	
Apixaban	Eliquis
Heparin	Heparin Sodium Add-Vantage
Fondaparinux	Arixtra
Argatroban	Acova
Antiplatelets	
Acetyl Salicylic Acid	Aspirin, Ascriptin, Durlaza, Ecotrin, Ecpirin, Fasprin, Halfprin, Miniprin
Dipyridamole/Aspirin	Aggrenox
Clopidogrel	Plavix
Ticlopidine	Ticlid
Abciximab	Reopro
Low–Molecular Weight Heparins	
Ardeparin	Indeparin
Dalteparin	Fragmin
Enoxaparin	Lovenox, Thrombiflo, Cutenox
Thrombolytic	
Alteplase	Activase, tissue plasminogen activator (tPA)
Diabetes Control Agents	
Insulin Products	
Insulin Lispro	Humalog
Insulin Aspart	Novolog
Insulin Glulisine	Apidra
Insulin Regular	—
Insulin NPH	—
Insulin Detemir	Levemir
Insulin Glargine	Lantus
Non-Insulin Injectable Agents	
Pramlintide	Symlin
Exenatide	Byetta
Liraglutide	Victoza

(*continued*)

(continued)

Generic Name	Trade Name
Diabetes Control Agents (*continued*)	
Dulaglutide	Trulicity
Albiglutide	Tanzeum
Oral Agents	
Glipizide	Glucotrol
Glyburide	Micronase
Glimepiride	Amaryl
Metformin	Glucophage
Pioglitazone	Actos
Sitagliptin	Januvia
Linagliptin	Tradjenta
Saxagliptin	Onglyza
Nateglinide	Starlix
Repaglinide	Prandin
Miglitol	Glyset
Acarbose	Precose
Tolazamide	Tolinase
Tolbutamide	Orinase
Intracranial Pressure–Reducing Agents	
Hypertonic saline	3%, 7.5%, 23.4%
Mannitol	Osmitrol, Resectisol, Aridol
Lipid-Lowering Agents	
Bile Acid Sequestrants	
Colestipol	Colestid
Cholestyramine	Questran
Colesevelam	Welchol
Cholesterol Absorption Inhibitor	
Ezetimibe	Zetia
Fibric Acid Derivatives	
Gemfibrozil	Lopid
Fenofibrate	Tricor

(continued)

(continued)

Generic Name	Trade Name
Lipid-Lowering Agents (*continued*)	
Nicotinic Acid	
Niacin	Niacin-SR, Niacor, Niaspan ER, Slo-Niacin
Statins	
Simvastatin	Zocor
Atorvastatin	Lipitor
Lovastatin	Mevacor
Rosuvastatin	Crestor
Pravastatin	Pravachol
Fluvastatin	Lescol
Pitavastatin	Livalo
Icosapent ethyl	Vascepa
Omega-3 Fatty Acids	
Omega-e ethyl esters	Lovaza
Neuroleptics	
Haloperidol	Haldol
Aripiprazole	Abilify
Quetiapine	Seroquel
Risperidone	Risperdal
Olanzapine	Zyprexa
Ziprasidone	Geodon
Neurostimulants	
Methylphenidate	Ritalin, Concerta, Daytrana
Dextroamphetamine	Dexedrine
Amantadine	Symmetrel
Carbidopa/levodopa	Sinemet, Parcopa
Donepezil	Aricept
Bromocriptine	Parlodel
Sedatives	
Propofol	Diprivan

(continued)

(continued)

Generic Name	Trade Name
Sedatives (*continued*)	
Midazolam	Versed
Lorazepam	Ativan
Dexmedetomidine	Precedex
Vasopressors and Inotropes	
Epinephrine	Adrenalin
Norepinephrine	Levophed
Phenylephrine	Neo-Synephrine
Dobutamine	Dobutrex
Dopamine	Intropin
Milrinone	Primacor
Vasopressin	Pitressin

Appendix B: Neuroscience Glossary

Agnosia—Failure to recognize stimuli when the appropriate sensory systems are functioning adequately; commonly occurs in visual, tactile, and auditory forms

Antithrombotics—Medications that prevent clot formation; two classes are anticoagulants and antiplatelet agents

Aphasia—Loss of ability to use language and to communicate thoughts verbally or in writing; receptive aphasia: inability to understand; expressive aphasia: inability to speak/write

Ataxia—Uncoordination or clumsiness of movement that is not the result of muscular weakness; it is caused by vestibular, cerebellar, or sensory disorders

Aura—Subjective sensation preceding a paroxysmal attack; may precede migraines or seizures and can be psychic or sensory in nature

Clonic—Alternating contraction and relaxation of muscles

Collateral circulation—Circulation of blood established through enlargement of minor vessels and anastomosis of vessels with those of adjacent parts when a major vein or artery is functionally impaired (as by obstruction)

Comorbid conditions—Presence of one or more disorders in addition to the primary disorder; for example, a stroke patient with diabetes and hypertension—these are comorbid conditions

Contralateral—Originating in, or affecting, the opposite side of the body

Decerebrate—Posture characterized by a rigid—possibly arched—spine, rigidly extended arms and legs, and plantar flexion; indicative of a brainstem lesion

Decorticate—Posture characterized by a rigid spine, inwardly flexed arms, extended and internally rotated legs, and plantar flexion; indicative of a brainstem lesion

Delirium—Mental confusion and excitement characterized by disorientation for time and place, usually with illusions and hallucinations; possible causes are fever, shock, exhaustion, anxiety, or drug overdose

Dementia—An acquired, generalized, and often progressive impairment of cognitive function that affects the content, but not the level, of consciousness; may indicate pathology affecting the cerebral cortex, its subcortical connections, or both

Diplopia—Double vision; may indicate pathology involving the cranial nerves, eyeballs, cerebellum, cerebrum, or meninges

Dissection—Separation of the layers of an arterial or venous wall resulting in reduced lumen and possibly complete occlusion

Dysphagia—Difficulty swallowing or inability to swallow

Dysphasia—Impaired ability to communicate with verbal or written language; seldom used in clinical care, as aphasia has come to be used to represent not only the inability to communicate, but also the impaired ability to communicate; dysphasia is often confused with dysphagia

Fissure—Deep cleft or groove between segments of the cerebral cortex; larger than a sulcus

Gray matter—Largest portion of the brain; neuronal cell bodies and glial cells in the cortex and deep nuclei process information originating in the sensory organs or in other gray matter regions

Gyrus (plural is **gyri**)—Prominent convolutions on the surface of the cerebral hemispheres

Hemianopia—Loss of half of the visual field; homonymous hemianopia means that both right visual fields or both left visual fields are lost

Hemiparesis—Weakness affecting only one side of the body; may indicate an intracranial structural lesion

Hemiplegia—Paralysis affecting only one side of the body; may indicate pathology of upper motor neurons

Hemorrhagic transformation—Also called hemorrhagic conversion; that is, leakage of blood from vessels in the ischemic stroke bed; the presence of blood "transforms" an ischemic stroke into a hemorrhagic stroke on imaging, but improved imaging makes it possible to differentiate a primary hemorrhage from an ischemic stroke with hemorrhagic transformation

Hyperreflexia—Abnormally intense response to a stimulus; may indicate a lesion of the upper motor neurons and suggests lack of cortical control over the reflex

Ictal—Pertaining to or caused by a sudden attack such as acute epilepsy

Infarction—Irreversible damage or death of tissue

Intima—Innermost lining of an artery or vein

Intrathecal—Introduction of substance into the subarachnoid space of the brain or spinal cord; certain drugs are given this way to avoid the blood–brain barrier

Ipsilateral—Originating in or affecting the same side of the body

Ischemia—Insufficient blood flow to meet metabolic demand; if not corrected, leads to hypoxia and infarction

Myelin—White fatty material that encloses the axons of myelinated nerve fibers; acts as an insulator, increasing the speed of transmission of nerve signals

Myoclonic—Twitching or clonic spasm of a muscle or group of muscles

Nerve palsy—Neurological defect caused by dysfunction of the nerve that controls that part of the body; for example, third cranial nerve palsy is manifested by limited eye movements and ptosis

Nystagmus—Involuntary, rhythmic, oscillating motions of the eyes

Parenchyma—Functional tissue of an organ, distinguished from connective and supporting tissue

Plateau—Point in recovery when progress slows or stops; often used as criterion for discontinuing therapy services

Postictal—Phase that follows an attack such as acute epilepsy; subjective sensation can be variable

Ptosis—Drooping eyelid

Recanalization—Restoration of blood flow to an arterial occlusion site

Spasticity—Unusual tightness, or stiffness, of muscle due to increased tone, or hypertonia; occurs within days to weeks in 30% of stroke patients

Sulcus (plural is **sulci**)—Deep grooves on the surface of the cerebral hemisphere

Supratentorial—Refers to portions of the brain above the tentorium (*see* Tentorium)

Symmetry—Two sides having the same size and shape

Tentorium—Extension of the dura mater that separates the cerebellum from the inferior portion of the occipital lobes

Thrombolysis—Dissolution, or lysis, of a blood clot

Tonic—Pertaining to, or characterized by, tension or contraction, especially muscular tension

Ventricles—Four hollow spaces in the brain that are filled with cerebrospinal fluid

Vertigo—Sensation of moving around in space, or having objects move around the person; indicates disturbance of the equilibratory apparatus

White matter—Bundles of myelinated axons that connect various gray matter areas of the brain and carry nerve impulses between neurons

Appendix C: List of National Stroke Care Guidelines

There are numerous national guidelines related to stroke care. This is a list of the most common ones used by certified Stroke Centers.

AANN Clinical Practice Guidelines—available online: www.aann.org

American Heart Association/American Stroke Association Focused Update of the 2013 Guidelines for the Early Management of Patients With Acute Ischemic Stroke Regarding Endovascular Treatment: A Guideline for Healthcare Professionals From the American Heart Association/American Stroke Association (2015)

American Heart Association/American Stroke Association Guidelines—available online for free: strokeassociation.org

Care of the Patient With Aneurysmal Subarachnoid Hemorrhage. (2012). AANN clinical practice guideline series

Comprehensive Overview of Nursing and Interdisciplinary Rehabilitation Care of the Stroke Patient: A Scientific Statement From the American Heart Association (2010)

Evidence for Stroke Family Caregiver and Dyad Interventions: A Statement for Healthcare Professionals From the American Heart Association/American Stroke Association (2014)

Expansion of the Time Window for Treatment of Acute Ischemic Stroke With Intravenous Tissue Plasminogen Activator: A Science Advisory From the American Heart Association/American Stroke Association (2009)

Guidelines for Adult Stroke Rehabilitation and Recovery: A Guideline for Healthcare Professionals From the American Heart Association/American Stroke Association (2015)

Guidelines for the Early Management of Patients With Acute Ischemic Stroke: A Guideline for Healthcare Professionals From the American Heart Association/American Stroke Association (2013)

Guidelines for the Management of Aneurysmal Subarachnoid Hemorrhage: A Guideline for Healthcare Professionals From the American Heart Association/American Stroke Association (2012)

Guidelines for the Management of Spontaneous Intracerebral Hemorrhage: A Guideline for Healthcare Professionals From the American Heart Association/American Stroke Association (2015)

Guidelines for the Prevention of Stroke in Patients With Stroke and Transient Ischemic Attack: A Guideline for Healthcare Professionals From the American Heart Association/American Stroke Association (2014)

Guidelines for the Prevention of Stroke in Women: A Guideline for Healthcare Professionals From the American Heart Association/American Stroke Association (2014)

Guidelines for the Primary Prevention of Stroke: A Statement for Healthcare Professionals From the American Heart Association/American Stroke Association (2014)

Interactions Within Stroke Systems of Care: A Policy Statement From the American Heart Association/American Stroke Association (2013)

Palliative Care and Cardiovascular Disease and Stroke: A Policy Statement for Healthcare Professionals From the American Heart Association/American Stroke Association (2016)

Recommendations for the Implementation of Telemedicine Within Stroke Systems of Care: A Policy Statement From the American Heart Association (2009)

Recommendations for the Management of Cerebral and Cerebellar Infarction and Swelling: A Statement for Healthcare Professionals From the American Heart Association/American Stroke Association (2014)

Scientific Rationale for the Inclusion and Exclusion Criteria for Intravenous Alteplase in Acute Ischemic Stroke: A Statement for Healthcare Professionals From the American Heart Association/American Stroke Association (2015)

Telemedicine Quality and Outcomes in Stroke: A Scientific Statement for Healthcare Professionals From the American Heart Association/American Stroke Association (2016)

Index

postcentral gyrus, 14, 22
posterior fossa, 21
poststroke spasticity, contractures, 115,
    120
postural hypotension, 84, 96
preventive care
    antithrombotic treatment, PFO, 32, 38
    ARIC study, 36
    atrial fibrillation, 27, 34
        anticoagulation resumption, 33, 38
        CHADS$_2$ score, 27, 34
        long-term implantable monitors, 32,
            37–38
        self-assessment, 28, 35
    community education, 31, 37
    Crispus Attucks community center,
        33, 38
    empathy, 140, 145
    home medications, 139, 145
    hypertension control and statin
        therapy, 37
    INTERSTROKE study, 29, 35–36
    physical activity, 30, 37
    primordial prevention, 34
    right-sided carotid artery stenosis,
        32, 37
    risk factors, 35–36
    secondary prevention, 35
    smoking cessation, 28, 35
    speech and occupational therapy, 141,
        146
    stroke education, 33, 38
    stroke incidence, 29, 36
    support for caregiver, 31, 37
    tertiary prevention, 35
    TIA and CEA, 27–28, 35
    type 2 diabetes and hypertension, 27,
        34
Primary Stroke Center (PSC), 125, 128
PSC. See Primary Stroke Center
pure motor syndromes, 23

recanalization, 97
recreational therapists, 118
reperfusion syndrome, 81, 95
right parietal lobe infarcts, 82, 95
right-sided carotid artery stenosis, 32, 37

rivaroxaban (Xarelto), 102, 109
root cause analysis, 126, 129

SAH. See subarachnoid hemorrhage
SCRN® certification exam. See Stroke
    Certified Registered Nurse
    certification exam
sedatives, 152–153
sensory strip, 21
SIADH. See syndrome of inappropriate
    antidiuretic hormone
skilled nursing facility (SNF), 114, 119
SLP. See speech and language
    pathologist
smoking cessation, 28, 35
SNF. See skilled nursing facility
spatial extinction, 115, 119
speech and language pathologist (SLP),
    83–84, 96
statins, 152
stenosis and transient ischemic attack
    (TIA), 27, 35
stroke
    community education, 31, 37
    high cholesterol, 30, 36–37
    incidence, 29, 36
    nursing care
        certification, 3–4
        history, 1–2
        leadership role in, 3
    physical activity, 30, 37
    positive family history, 30, 36
Stroke Belt, 53–54, 61
stroke center certification, 126, 129
Stroke Certified Registered Nurse
    (SCRN®) certification exam
    administration, 7
    application process canceling, 8
    appointment postponing, 8
    appointment rescheduling, 8
    appointment scheduling, 7
    categories, 6–7
    vs. CNRN, 9–10
    day of, 10–11
    eligibility criteria, 5–6
    format, 6
    night before, 10

notification of results, 7
passing score, 9
score maximization, 10
stroke databases, 124, 128
stroke diagnostics
Brain Attack Coalition's
recommendations, 66, 72
cerebral angiography, 66, 69, 72, 73
chest x-ray, 68, 73
CT angiogram, 64, 66, 68–70, 72, 73
CT imaging, 64, 67, 68, 70, 72, 73
echocardiogram, 64, 71
implantable cardiac monitor, 65, 71
IV tPA administration, 63, 70
MRI imaging, 67, 72
MRI/MRA, 64, 71
noncontrast CT, 67, 72
transcranial Doppler ultrasonography,
66, 68, 72, 73
transesophageal echocardiogram,
64–65, 71
video fluoroscopic swallowing exam,
65, 71
subacute rehabilitation facility, 114, 119
subarachnoid hemorrhage (SAH), 13, 21,
23, 65, 71
complications, 78, 93
education, 89, 99
lumbar puncture, 65, 71
noncontrast CT, 67, 72
normothermia maintainance, 135,
144
oral nimodipine, 107, 111
oxygenation, 81, 95
postaneurysm repair, 136, 144
postintervention environment, 136,
144
rebleeding risk, 135, 144
vasospasm
Hunt and Hess score, 135, 144
monitoring, 66, 72
nimodipine, 135, 144
risk, 82, 96
syndrome of inappropriate antidiuretic
hormone (SIADH), 80, 95
systems and quality care
benchmarking, 123, 127

Brain Attack Coalition's
recommendations, 66, 72, 123, 127
clinical practice guidelines, 125, 128
Comprehensive Stroke Center, 125,
128
NIHSS certification, 124, 128
Plan, Do, Study, Act (PDSA) process,
124, 128
Primary Stroke Center, 125, 128
root cause analysis, 126, 129
stroke databases, 124, 128
stroke unit benefits, 125, 128

telemedicine, 44, 57
temporal lobe, 14, 22
temporal lobe stroke, 96
tentorium, 13, 21
thalamus, 14, 22
therapeutic cooling and shivering, 107,
111
thrombolysis in cerebral infarction
(TICI) score, 133, 143
TIA. *See* transient ischemic attack
TICI score. *See* thrombolysis in cerebral
infarction score
tPA. *See* IV tissue plasminogen activator
(tPA)
transesophageal echocardiogram,
64, 71
transient ischemic attack (TIA)
ABCD$_2$ score, 76, 91
CT and MRI imaging, 67, 72
education, 52–53, 60, 88, 99
improved CT and MRI imaging, 126,
129
tunica intima, 18, 24

upper extremity and gait training
plan of care, 139, 145
reducing muscle strength, 138, 145
shoulder subluxation, 138, 145
treadmill training, 139, 145
urinary tract infection (UTI)
poststroke, 85, 97
risk for, 85, 97
U.S. State Board Test Pool Exam, 5
UTI. *See* urinary tract infection

INDEX